Normal Findings in Radiographgy

Torsten B. Moeller, M.D.

Am Caritas-Krankenhaus
Dillingen/Saar
Germany

190 Illustrations

Thieme
Stuttgart · New York 2000

Library of Congress Cataloging-in-Publication Data

Moeller, Torsten B.
  [Roentgennormalbefunde. English.]
  Normal findings in radiography / Torsten B. Moeller
      p. cm.
  Translation of the 2nd German ed.
  Includes bibliographical references and index.
  ISBN 0-86577-871-X – ISBN 3-13-116531-6
  1. Radiography, Medical. 2. Reference values (Medicine). 3. Human anatomy. I. Title.
  [DNLM: 1. Radiography. WN 200 M726r 1999a]
  RC78.M5913   1999
  616.07'572–dc21   99-040799

Translated by Terry Telger, Ft. Worth, TX, USA

This book is an authorized revised and expanded translation of the 2nd German edition published and copyrighted 1996 by Georg Thieme Verlag, Stuttgart, Germany. Title of the German edition: Röntgennormalbefunde

© 2000 Georg Thieme Verlag,
Rüdigerstrasse 14,
D-70469 Stuttgart, Germany
Thieme New York, 333 Seventh Avenue,
New York, NY 10001, USA

Typesetting by primustype R. Hurler GmbH, D-73274 Notzingen, Germany
typeset on Textline/HerculesPro
Cover design by Cyclus, Stuttgart
Printed in Germany by
Offizin Andersen Nexö, Leipzig

ISBN 3-13-116531-6 (GTV)
ISBN 0-86577-871-X (TNY)   1 2 3 4 5 6

For my parents,
Alfred and Friedel Moeller,
and for Barbara

Preface

This book deals with the apparently banal subject of normal radiographic findings: while the normal is common, it is not always simple. Anyone who has ever had occasion to read radiographic films has experienced the difficulties inherent in systematically interpreting images and formulating the findings. This book addresses three questions that are basic to radiographic interpretation:

— What system should I follow in reading an image, and how can I tell if the findings are normal?
— How do I formulate the findings?
— What quantitative parameters can I use to confirm normality, and how do I measure them?

Normal Findings in Radiography follows a rigorous format in which a brief description of normal findings is followed by a checklist that recapitulates the sequence of the descriptive text and provides a systematic framework for image interpretation. For clarity, similar phrasing is used in the textual descriptions and the checklists. Most sections conclude with a table of "Important Data" listing the normal ranges of values for the most important measurable parameters, which are highlighted on illustrative radiographs.

The sample descriptions of normal radiographic findings in the text portions of the book can serve only as guidelines, which must be tailored according to whether the case requires a gross assessment or a detailed evaluation. In all cases, however, the cornerstones of a quality x-ray report remain the same: simplicity, clarity, and precision. I hope that this book will serve as a guide for radiologists, especially those in training, in the routine interpretation of x-ray films.

Summer 1999   *Torsten B. Moeller*

Contents

The Skull

Skull, Biplane Views

The calvaria is normal in shape, thickness, and size. There are no abnormalities of mineralization or bone structure. The contours of the calvaria are smooth and sharp with no abnormal defects or discontinuities. The cranial sutures appear normal for age. There is no sign of abnormal calcifications.

The skull base presents a normal anatomical configuration and smooth borders, with a normal appearance of the planum sphenoidale, sella turcica, and posterior cranial fossa. Imaged portions of the facial skeleton and upper cervical spine are normally developed and have smooth, sharp contours. Evaluable portions of the paranasal sinuses are unremarkable.

Imaged soft tissues show no abnormalities.

Interpretation

The skull appears normal.

Checklist

Shape, size	• Approximately hemispherical
	• Dimensions (see below)
Thickness	• Normal bone thickness (see below)
	• Three layers (inner table, diploë, outer table)
Structure	• Mineralization
	• No circumscribed densities (sharp or indistinct, cloudy, striate, patchy)
	• No circumscribed areas of decalcification or erosion (rounded, oblong, with sclerosis? fracture lines? sharp or indistinct?)
	• Convolutional markings regular, not increased
Vascular channels	• Arteries, diploic veins, emissary veins: course, shape, thickness, caliber, location
Contours	• Outer and inner tables are smooth and sharp
	• No defects or discontinuities
	• No spicules or excrescences
Cranial sutures	• Course
	• Open or closed? (see below)
Cranial cavity	• Calcifications? (If so: location—e.g., pineal body: centered, not displaced)
Skull base	• Normal configuration (see below)
	• Anterior, middle, and posterior cranial fossae
	• No enlargement of sella
Facial skeleton	• Frontal sinuses (anatomy, pneumatization)
	• Nasal cavity (width, aeration, septum on the midline)
	• Orbital roof and sidewalls intact
Cervical spine	• Position
	• Tip of dens (see below)
Soft tissues	• Intact soft-tissue coverage
	• No swelling or foreign bodies

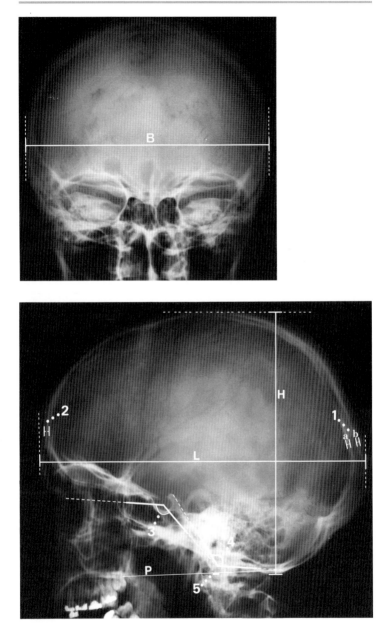

Important Data

Cranial dimensions:

$$\frac{1 \, [\text{Length (L)} + \text{width (W)} + \text{height (H)} \, (\text{in cm})]}{3}$$

= 16.3–19.5 (15.7–19.5 in women).

Normal values: length 21.2 cm, width 16.8 cm, height 15.6 cm (in women: L 20.1 cm, W 16.2 cm, H 15.1 cm).

1. Calvarial thickness:

(a) Inner table = ca. 0.5 mm; (b) outer table = ca. 1.5 mm

2. Total thickness of frontal cortex = ca. 1.5 mm

(The above values are only approximate owing to marked inter- and intraindividual variations: e.g., the thinnest areas are the orbital roof, temporal squama, and the glenoid fossa of the TMJ; the thickest area, at 3–8 mm, is the parietal tuber.)

Cranial sutures: All sutures are closed by age 20 years; one of the first to close is the frontal suture (by age 3), the last is the spheno-occipital synchondrosis (by age 20); ossification is complete by about age 40.

Skull base:

3. Base angle (nasion–sellar tubercle–basion) = 123°–152°

4. Boogard's angle (between foramen magnum and clivus) = 119–135°

5. Relation of cervical spine to skull base: the tip of the dens projects no more than 5 mm past the palato-occipital line (P).

Occipital View

The imaged portions of the calvaria are normal in shape, thickness, and symmetry. The lambdoid suture and other imaged cranial sutures are normal for age and display a normal course. They show proper bone structure and mineralization. The calvaria presents smooth, sharp outlines with no abnormal contour defects or fracture lines. The foramen magnum is normal in its shape, width, and margins. The cranial cavity is unremarkable. The soft tissues show no abnormalities.

Interpretation

The occiput and foramen magnum appear normal.

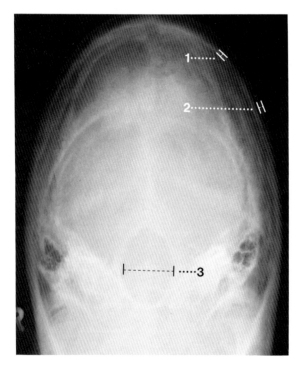

Checklist

Shape	• Symmetrical
Sutures	• Lambdoid suture and parts of the sagittal suture: open or closed (by age 18 years)
	• Normal course
	• No increased sclerosis
	• Wormian bones? (e.g., interparietal bone)
Structure	• Mineralization
	• Sharp delineation of bony structures
	• No circumscribed lucencies or densities (with or without sclerosis)
	• No fracture lines
	• Vascular channels: arteries, diploic and emissary veins (course variable, not always symmetrical, same approximate size)
Contours	• Outer and inner tables smooth and sharp
	• Width (see below)
	• No contour defects or discontinuities
	• No exostoses or bony excrescences
	• No periosteal elevation
Foramen magnum	• Shape (oval, symmetrical)
	• Width (see below)
	• Smooth, sharp inner contours
	• No discontinuities
Cranial cavity	• Calcifications? (If so: location)
Soft tissues	• Intact
	• No swelling
	• Calcifications? (Location)
	• No foreign bodies

Important Data

1. Thickness of inner table: ca. 0.5 cm
2. Thickness of outer table: ca. 1.5 mm
3. Diameter of foramen magnum: ca. 3.5 mm
(Caution: projection errors!)

Paranasal Sinuses

The paranasal sinuses and nasal cavity are normally shaped and symmetrically disposed. The nasal septum is centered on the midline. The sinuses show normal pneumatization and lucency, and their contours are smooth and sharply defined.

Imaged portions of the facial skeleton are unremarkable. There are no radiopaque foreign bodies.

Interpretation

The nasal cavities and paranasal sinuses appear normal.

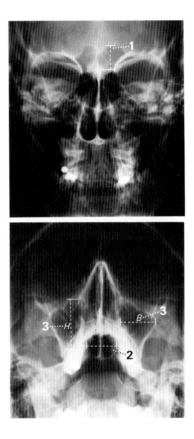

Checklist

Shape, size	• Frontal sinus (see below)
	• Ethmoid cells
	• Sphenoid sinus
	• Maxillary sinuses (see below)
	• Nasal cavity: symmetry, nasal septum centered
Pneumati-zation	• Radiolucency (symmetrical except for frontal sinuses)
	• No sinus clouding
	• No air–fluid levels
Contours	• Smooth and sharp
	• No contour defects
	• No circumscribed cortical thinning or thickening
	• No expansion
Other bony structures	• Facial skeleton, orbits, petrous ridges:
	— Shape (symmetry)
	— Structure
	— Contours (radiolucent lines)
Soft tissues	• No foreign bodies or calcifications
	• No swelling

Important Data

1. Frontal sinus: height = ca. 1.5–2 cm
2. Sphenoid sinus: width = 0.9–1.4 cm
3. Maxillary sinuses: width (W) and height (H) = ca. 2 cm

Orbits, Posteroanterior View

The imaged portions of the facial skeleton are reasonably symmetrical.
They show normal anatomical development with proper bone structure
and mineralization. The bony orbital margins have smooth, sharp con-
tours. The superior orbital fissure shows a normal configuration.
Imaged portions of the paranasal sinuses show no abnormalities.
The petrous ridges are unremarkable in their shape and contours.
There are no soft-tissue swellings or radiopaque foreign bodies.

Interpretation

Both orbits appear normal.

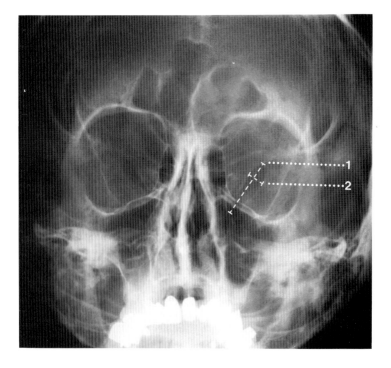

Checklist

Superior orbital fissure Shape	• Symmetrical
	• Course
	• Length (see below)
	• Width (see below)
	• Margins (no circumscribed expansion)
Contours	• Cortex smooth and sharp (orbital floor, sidewalls, and roof)
	• No contour defects or discontinuities
	• No sclerosis
	• No circumscribed expansion
Structure	• Mineralization
	• No circumscribed lucencies or expansions
	• No densities
Paranasal sinuses	• Frontal sinus, ethmoid cells, upper part of maxillary sinuses:
	— Shape
	— Pneumatization
	— Radiolucency: clouding, fluid levels
	— Smooth, intact bony contours
Petrous pyramids	• Petrous ridges:
	— Shape
	— Symmetry
	— Smooth, sharp contours
Soft tissues	• No intraocular foreign bodies (shape, location)
	• No swelling
	• No calcifications

Important Data

Superior orbital fissure:
1. Length = 15 mm
2. Maximum width = 5 mm

Orbit, Oblique Rhese View

The bony boundaries of the orbit are normally shaped and sharply de-lineated with no contour defects. The optic canal is normal in position and diameter.

Other imaged skeletal structures are unremarkable in their shape, bony structure, and mineralization.

Imaged portions of the paranasal sinuses appear normal.

There are no radiopaque foreign bodies.

Interpretation

The orbit and optic canal appear normal.

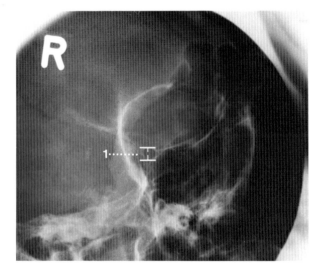

Checklist

Shape	• Orbital roof
	• Orbital sidewalls
	• Orbital floor
	• Optic canal (see below)
Contours	• Cortex smooth and sharp
	• No contour defects or discontinuities
	• No sclerosis
Structure	• Mineralization
	• No circumscribed lucencies or expansions
	• No densities
Paranasal sinuses	• Posterior ethmoid cells, portions of the frontal and maxillary sinuses, sphenoid sinus:
	— Good pneumatization
	— No clouding
	— No fluid levels
	— Smooth, intact bony contours
Other skeletal structures	• Sphenoid wing
	• Planum sphenoidale
	• Zygoma (if evaluable)
Soft tissues	• Intraocular foreign bodies
	• No swelling
	• No calcifications

Important Data

1. Diameter of optic canal = ca. 4–5 mm

Maxilla

The maxilla is normal in shape, symmetry, and size. It displays proper bone structure and mineralization. The outer bone structure is intact, with no pathological contour defects or radiolucent lines. The maxillary dentition appears normal.

Imaged portions of the facial skeleton, especially about the nose and paranasal sinuses, are unremarkable.

The soft tissues are free of swelling, radiopaque foreign bodies, and other abnormalities.

Interpretation

The maxilla and evaluable portions of the facial skeleton appear normal.

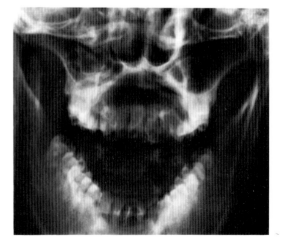

Checklist

Shape	• Elliptical
	• Symmetry, width (atrophy?) (the lateral portions of the maxilla are difficult to evaluate due to superimposed structures)
Structure	• Mineralization (cancellous bone usually is not demarcated)
	• No densities
	• No lucencies or fracture lines
Contours	• Intact with no discontinuities
	• Smooth, sharp margins
Dentition	• Normal number of teeth (see below)
	• No supernumerary or unerupted teeth
	• No persistent deciduous teeth
	• Intact restorations (crowns, bridges)
Rest of facial skeleton	• Orbits
	• Paranasal sinuses (frontal sinus and orbital roof, depending on collimation)
	• Nasal cavity
	• Zygoma and zygomatic arch
	• Imaged articular portions of the maxilla:
	— Shape
	— Structure
	— Contours (smooth, intact, no discontinuities)
	— Aeration (mucosal swelling, mass?)
Soft tissues	• Intact
	• No swelling
	• No calcifications (salivary glands)
	• No foreign bodies
	• No cutaneous emphysema

Important Data

1. Permanent dentition (if evaluable): 14 teeth + 2 wisdom teeth

Mandible, Clementschitsch View

The mandible is normal in shape, size, and symmetry. The mandibular condyles have a normal, symmetrical shape and position. They show proper bone structure and mineralization. The cortex is of normal thickness and presents smooth, sharp contours. The temporomandibular joint has normal contours. The mandibular dentition is normal. Evaluable portions of the maxilla and facial skeleton are unremarkable.

The soft tissues are normal with no signs of swelling, radiopaque foreign bodies, or calcifications.

Interpretation

The mandible and mandibular dentition appear normal. Evaluable portions of the maxilla and facial skeleton also appear normal.

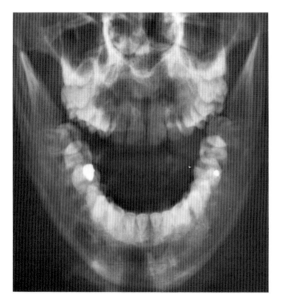

Checklist

Shape	• Mandible (elliptical), maxilla, maxillary sinuses, nasal cavity (septum centered), zygoma: symmetrical
	• Width of the mandible (hypertrophy, atrophy)
	• Mandibular condyles (anatomy, position) symmetrical
Mandible Structure	• Mineralization
	• Cancellous bone sharply delineated
	• Normal trabeculation of the cancellous bone
	• No circumscribed densities or lucencies (e.g., cystlike lucency, possibly with sclerotic margins; fracture lines)
Contours	• Cortex smooth and sharp, shows uniform thickness
	— No circumscribed thickening or thinning
	• No contour defects or discontinuities
	• No periosteal reaction or elevation
	• Mandibular canal (inferior alveolar nerve):
	— Smooth walls, no discontinuities, normal diameter
	• Mandibular condyle and articular tubercle:
	— Shape, position
	— Smooth contours, no destructive changes
	— Normal width of joint space
	— No calcifications or foreign bodies
Other skeletal structures	• Maxilla (particularly the anterior part)
Structure	• Mineralization
	• No increased density or lucency (fracture?)
Contours	• Intact with no defects or discontinuities
	• Borders smooth and sharp
	• No circumscribed thinning or expansion
Dentition	• Only the anterior maxillary teeth can be evaluated (number, position, restorations)
Soft tissues	• Intact, no swelling, calcification (e.g., salivary glands, intra-articular and periarticular), foreign bodies
	• No clouding of maxillary sinuses or nasal cavity

Important Data

Permanent mandibular dentition: 14 teeth and 2 wisdom teeth

Ramus of the Mandible

The imaged portion of the mandible is unremarkable in shape and size, with a normal-appearing mandibular angle. They show proper bone structure and mineralization. The cortex has a normal thickness with smooth, sharp contours and no abnormal contour defects.

The bones of the temporomandibular joint are normal in shape and position and have smooth contours. The dentition, including any dental work, is unremarkable.

There is no evidence of soft-tissue calcifications or radiopaque foreign bodies.

Interpretation

The mandibular ramus and temporomandibular joint appear normal.

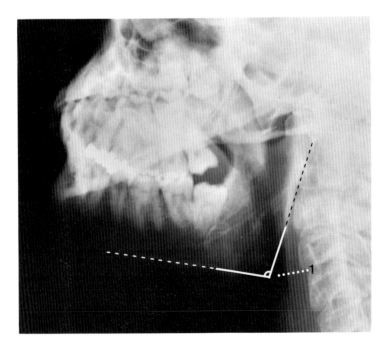

Checklist

Shape	• Width (hypertrophy, atrophy)
	• Mandibular angle (see below)
	• Configuration of the condylar and coronoid processes
Structure	• Mineralization
	• Cancellous bone is sharply delineated and shows a normal structural pattern
	• No densities or lucencies (e.g., cystlike lucency along the tooth root)
	• No widening of periodontal spaces
Contours	• Intact
	• Smooth, sharp borders
	• No contour defects or discontinuities
	• No circumscribed thinning or thickening
	• Mandibular canal: course, contours (smooth?)
Joint	• Smooth outline of mandibular condyle
	• Normal articulation of the condyle in the glenoid fossa
	• Articular tubercle: shape, contours (smooth)
Dentition	• Normal number of teeth (see below)
	• No supernumerary or unerupted teeth
	• No persistent deciduous teeth
	• Restorations (crowns, bridges)
	• Attachments of the teeth
	• In some studies: number and shape of the articulating maxillary teeth
Soft tissues	• Intact
	• No swelling
	• No calcifications (salivary glands, intra-articular and periarticular)
	• No foreign bodies

Important Data

1. Mandibular angle: ca. 110–140°
Permanent dentition in each hemimandible: 2 molars, 2 premolars, 1 canine, 2 incisors, 1 wisdom tooth

Orthopantomogram of the Maxillofacial Skull

The imaged portions of the maxilla, mandible, and facial skeleton are normal in shape and size. They show proper bone structure and mineralization. The cortical margins are smooth and sharply defined with no pathological contour defects. The nerve canal in the alveolar bone presents normal outlines.

Both temporomandibular joints appear normal and have joint spaces of normal width.

The dentition, including any dental work, is unremarkable. The teeth are normal in number, position, shape, and structure. The roots extend a normal distance into the alveolar bone, and there is no appreciable widening of the periodontal space.

The maxillary and other paranasal sinuses are clear and aerated and, like the orbital floor, have smooth walls.

There is no evidence of radiopaque foreign bodies or soft-tissue swelling.

Interpretation

The maxilla, mandible, and imaged portions of the facial skeleton appear normal.

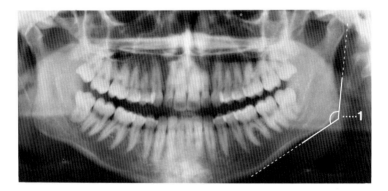

Important Data

1. Mandibular angle = 110–140°
Permanent dentition: 28 teeth and 4 wisdom teeth.

Checklist

Shape	• Orbits and zygomata: "eyeglass" configuration
	• Jaws: harmonious curve
	• Nose: septum straight and centered
	• Maxillary sinuses: symmetry, size
	• Temporomandibular joint and mandibular angle (see below)
Jaws	• Mineralization
Bone structure	• No circumscribed densities or lucencies (e.g., fracture lines, demineralized areas, radicular lucencies)
	• Sharp delineation of cancellous bone structure
	• No cystlike expansions (sclerotic margins)
Contours	• Cortex smooth and sharp, shows uniform thickness
	• No circumscribed thickening or thinning
	• No contour defects or discontinuities
	• No periosteal reaction or elevation
	• Mandibular canal and foramen (inferior alveolar nerve):
	− Smooth, no discontinuities, normal width
	• Articular tubercle, glenoid fossa:
	− Shape, position, smooth contours (destruction?)
	− Normal width of joint space
	− No calcifications or foreign bodies
Dentition	• Number of teeth (see below)
	• No supernumerary, unerupted, or deciduous teeth
	• Position (roughly equidistant spacing, relation of upper molars to floor of maxillary sinus)
	• Intact crown and enamel
	• Normal width of pulp canal and pulp cavity
	• Smooth, sharp contours (no defects)
	• Roots buried to the tooth neck in the alveolar bone
	• No widening of the periodontal spaces
Skull	• Mineralization
Bone structure	• No circumscribed densities or lucencies (fracture lines)
Contours	• Orbital floor, zygoma, alveolar zygomatic crest, walls of maxillary sinuses, nasal cavity, zygomatic arch, external auditory canal:
	− Cortex smooth and sharp, intact
	− Uniform cortical bone thickness
Soft tissues	• Gingiva, maxillary sinus mucosa
	• No calcifications, foreign bodies, or swelling

Nasal Skeleton, Lateral View

The nasal bone displays an anatomically normal shape. The nasal and frontal bones meet at a normal angle and are separated by a normal-appearing frontonasal suture. They show proper bone structure and mineralization. The nasal skeleton presents a smooth, sharp outline with no pathological contour defects.

The soft-tissue envelope is intact and shows no circumscribed swelling or radiopaque foreign bodies.

Interpretation

The nasal skeleton appears normal.

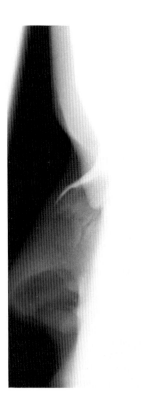

Checklist

Shape	•	Nasal bone
	•	Frontonasal suture
Position	•	Normal angle between the nasal and frontal bones (no abnormal upward or downward angulation)
Structure	•	Mineralization
	•	Bone structure
	•	No circumscribed densities or lucencies
	•	No expansion
Contours	•	Smooth, sharp outlines
	•	No abnormal defects (caution: sutures) or discontinuities
Soft tissues	•	Intact
	•	No swelling
	•	No radiopaque foreign bodies
	•	No calcifications

Zygomatic Arch

The zygomatic arch is normal in size and shape, with proper bone structure and mineralization. The cortical margins are smooth and sharp with no sign of abnormal contour defects. Other imaged portions of the facial skeleton are normally shaped and have sharp, smooth margins. The soft tissues are intact with no swelling, calcifications, or radiopaque foreign bodies.

Interpretation

The zygomatic arch appears normal.

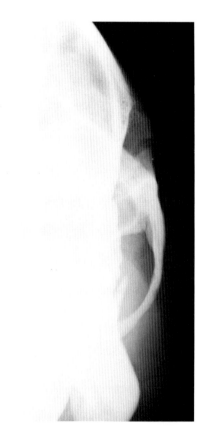

Checklist

Shape	•	A low arch, broadened at both ends
Structure	•	Mineralization
	•	No densities
	•	No lucencies
	•	No fracture line or cystic expansion
Contours	•	Smooth, sharp cortical margins
	•	No contour defects or discontinuities
Skull	•	Shape
	•	Bone structure
	•	Contours (calvaria, facial skeleton)
Soft tissues	•	Intact
	•	No swelling
	•	No calcifications or foreign bodies

Skull Base

The skull presents a normal, symmetrical shape. The nasal cavity and evaluable portions of the paranasal sinuses appear normal. The pharynx and nasopharynx are unremarkable. The bony portions of the middle cranial fossa are normal in their shape, structure, and boundaries. The neurovascular channels are properly positioned and have normal diameters. The mastoid cells are well pneumatized. The foramen magnum has a normal diameter. The calvaria presents a normal bone structure, and tangentially imaged portions have smooth margins and a normal thickness. The mandible and imaged soft-tissue structures are unremarkable.

Interpretation

The skull base appears normal.

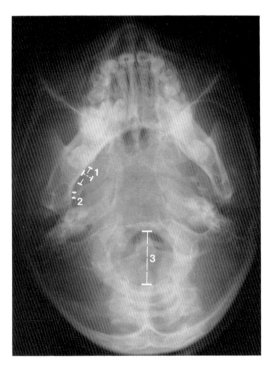

Checklist

Shape	• Skull shape
	• Symmetry (on an accurate projection)
Paranasal sinuses	• Maxillary sinuses (especially the posterior portion), sphenoid sinus
	• Ethmoid cells:
	— Shape
	— Smooth, intact wall contours (well delineated, no destruction), no wall thickening
	— Pneumatization (no soft-tissue opacity, no foreign bodies)
Nasal cavity	• Smooth, intact wall contours
	• Septum centered on the midline
	• No intranasal clouding or foreign bodies
Pharynx, nasopharynx	• Symmetrical, bulbous lucency
	• No circumscribed soft-tissue density
	• Smooth wall contours
Middle cranial fossa	• Sphenoid wings:
	— Bone structure (uniform throughout, no destruction)
	— Pterygoid and pterygopalatine fossae symmetrical on both sides
	— Smooth, intact wall contours
	— Normal width of foramina (see below)
	• Clivus:
	— Smooth, sharp borders
	— Symmetrical
	• Petrous pyramids:
	— Symmetry
	— Good pneumatization of the mastoid cells
	— No destructive changes
	— In some studies: posterior margin of petrous, internal porus acusticus
Other bony structures	• Foramen magnum
	• Calvaria (zygomatic arches)
	• Mandible (position, contours, structure)
Soft tissues	• No foreign bodies or calcifications

Important Data

Diameters of foramina:
1. **Foramen ovale: width = 3–7 mm, length = 5–11 mm**
2. **Foramen spinosum = 1–3.5 mm**
3. **Foramen magnum (by age 8 years) = ca. 3.5 cm**

Petrous Pyramids, Altschul Comparison View

Both petrous pyramids in this projection show symmetrical, anatomically normal development. Mineralization and bone structure are normal. The superior petrous ridges and normal-size internal acoustic meati present smooth, sharp margins on both sides. The inner ear structures are normal in shape and position. Both mandibular condyles and temporomandibular joints appear normal.

Other imaged portions of the skull display proper bone structure and mineralization.

The soft tissues are unremarkable and contain no radiopaque foreign bodies.

Interpretation

Both petrous pyramids and imaged portions of the cranial skeleton appear normal and symmetrical.

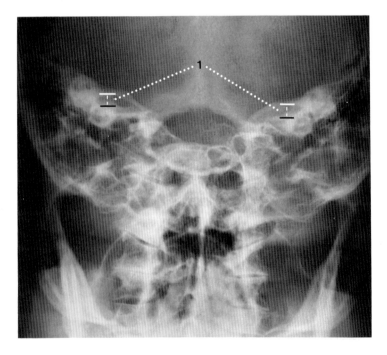

Checklist

Petrous pyramids	• Shape (wedge-shaped, symmetrical)
	• Position (parallel to skull base)
	• Structure (mineralization, pneumatization, no circumscribed densities or lucencies)
	• Contours (superior ridge: smooth, sharp, no defects or discontinuities)
Internal acoustic meatus	• Shape (symmetrical)
	• Luminal diameter (see below)
	• No circumscribed expansion, narrowing, or thickening
	• Contours (smooth, sharp)
	• No contour defects
Semicircular canals, cochlea, tympanic cavity	• Shape
	• Position
	• Symmetry
Mandibular condyles	• Shape (symmetry)
	• Position (centered)
	• Contours (smooth, sharp)
	• No contour defects
Styloid process	• Shape
	• Contours (smooth, sharp)
	• No contour defects
	• No calcifications
Other skeletal structures	• Shape
	• Structure (lucencies, densities, mineralization)
Soft tissues	• No swelling
	• No calcifications or foreign bodies

Important Data

1. *Internal acoustic meatus:*
   Diameter 5 mm (2–12 mm), maximum of 1 mm difference between the sides

Petrous Bone, Schüller View

The external and internal porus acusticus are well delineated and have smooth contours and normal luminal diameters. The boundaries of the mastoid are normal. The mastoid air cells are well pneumatized and show a normal arrangement and septal thickness. The contours of the Citelli angle are normal and intact. The sigmoid sinus presents a normal anterior contour.

The glenoid fossa, articular tubercle, and mandibular condyle are properly shaped and positioned and have smooth, sharp borders.

Interpretation

The mastoid and temporomandibular joint appear normal.

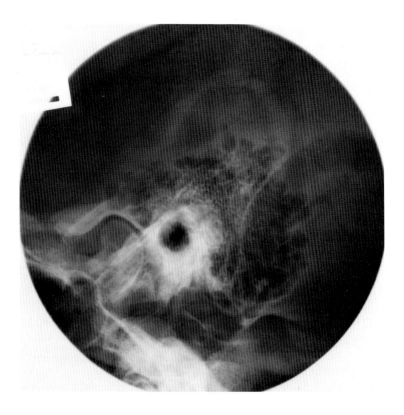

Checklist

Auditory canal	• Projection (see below)
	• Delineation
	• Smooth contours
	• Luminal diameter
	• No intraluminal mass
Mastoid	• Cellular anatomy (antrum, retrofacial cells, peritubal cells, peribulbar cells, marginal cells, terminal cells):
	• Cells are of mixed sizes, showing uniform enlargement from the antrum to the terminal cells
	• No cystlike expansion of cells (especially the terminal cells)
	• Pneumatization (no clouding of cells)
	• Normal septal thickness
Petrous pyramid	• Contours (superior ridge smooth and sharp)
	• No radiolucent lines
	• No radiolucent masses
	• No densities
	• Boundary of petrous pyramid with calvaria:
	— Citelli angle (= sinodural angle) shows no contour defects or erosion
	— Cells at the angle are clear and pneumatized
	• Sigmoid sinus (usually only the anterior border is seen):
	— Shape (S-shaped)
	— Position
	— Width (if evaluable)
Temporomandibular joint	• Glenoid fossa (shape, contour)
	• Articular tubercle (shape)
	• Mandibular condyle (shape, contour, position)
Soft tissues	• Foreign bodies, calcifications

Important Data

In an accurate Schüller projection, the internal and external acoustic meati are superimposed

Petrous Bone, Stenvers View

The imaged portions of the petrous bone and calvaria show a proper shape and position. The petrous bone structure is normal, and the petrous ridge presents a smooth contour. The internal porus acusticus and internal acoustic meatus have smooth, sharp borders with a normal luminal diameter. The superior and lateral semicircular canals have a normal shape. The imaged portion of the mastoid is well pneumatized. The occipital squama is unremarkable.

Interpretation

The petrous bone and internal auditory canal appear normal.

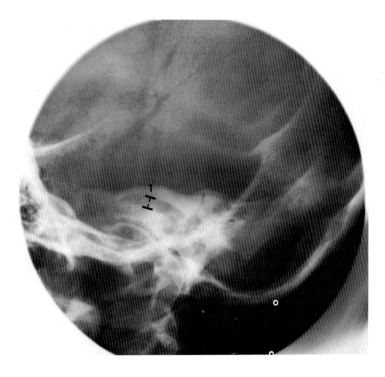

Checklist

Shape, position	●	Petrous bone, calvaria
Petrous bone	●	Bone structure (mineralization)
	●	Contours (petrous ridge and apex are smooth and sharp, no radiolucent lines, no discontinuities)
	●	No dense or lucent masses (especially in the medial part of the petrous pyramid)
	●	Pneumatization
	●	Facial canal (not expanded)
Internal Meatus and porus acusticus	●	Shape
	●	Position
	●	Luminal diameter (see below)
	●	Contours (smooth, sharp)
	●	No intraluminal mass
Inner ear	●	Superior and lateral semicircular canals visible
	●	Vestibule, cochlea
Mastoid cells and mastoid process	●	Cellular anatomy (small cells, cystlike expansion, e.g., in terminal cells?)
	●	Well pneumatized
	●	No clouding or fracture line
	●	Normal septal thickness
Calvaria	●	Occipital squama (structure, mineralization, no radiolucent lines)
Soft tissues	●	Foreign bodies?
	●	Calcifications?

Important Data

Internal acoustic meatus:
1. Diameter 5 mm (range 2–12 mm, right-left difference does not exceed 1 mm)
   Length 8 mm (range 4–25 mm, right-left difference does not exceed 2 mm)
   (May be difficult to measure in this projection)

Sella Turcica, Special View

The shape, position, and size of the sella are within normal limits. Mineralization and bone structure are normal. The cortex is of normal thickness and has sharp, smooth margins. The sphenoid sinus is normally aerated and shows no clouding. There are no intracranial calcium deposits.

Interpretation

The sella turcica appears normal.

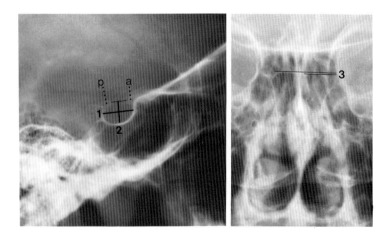

Checklist

Shape	• Depth and length of sella (see below) • No circumscribed ballooning or excavation of the sellar floor • No significant height discrepancy between the right and left sides (see below) • No erosion of the dorsum sellae or sphenoid sinus posterior wall • Normal inclination of the anterior (a) and posterior (p) clinoid process
Structure	• Mineralization • No circumscribed densities • No lucencies or expansions
Contours	• Cortex (smooth, sharp, normal thickness) • No thinning, impression, or bulging • No contour defects or discontinuities • No double contours (on an accurate projection!)
Sphenoid sinus	• Shape • Contours • Pneumatization (no opacities) • No foreign bodies
Neurocranium	• Intracranial calcium deposits (location?)

Important Data

Sella turcica:
1. Length = 5–16 mm
2. Depth = 4–12 mm

Floor of sella (posteroanterior projection):
3. Height discrepancy between right and left sides = less than 2 mm

The Spine

Full-Length Anteroposterior View

The cervical spine, thoracic spine, and lumbar spine show a normal position with a minimal degree of right–left–right convex scoliosis and normal vertebral alignment. The vertebral bodies are normal in their number, shape, size, and interrelationships. They show no abnormalities of mineralization or bone structure. The cortical margins of the vertebrae, including the end plates, are smooth and sharply defined.
The pedicles and transverse processes show a normal configuration. The disk spaces and spinal canal have normal diameters.
Imaged portions of the ribs are unremarkable.
The imaged soft tissues contain no radiopaque foreign bodies.

Interpretation

There is minimal right–left–right convex scoliosis of the spine with no abnormal findings.

Checklist

Position	● Scoliosis angle (see below)
Vertebrae number	● Normal vertebral and segmental alignment
	● 7 cervical, 12 thoracic, 5 lumbar
	● No short or supernumerary ribs
Shape	● Rectangular shape, height, size
	● No shortened or wedged vertebrae
Structure	● Mineralization
	● No patchy or linear densities or lucencies
Contours	● Cortex, including end plates, is smooth and sharp
	● No contour defects (impressions)
	● No sclerosis
	● No marginal osteophytes
Pedicles	● Elliptical, paired, symmetrical
Processes	● Spinous processes (alignment, deformity?)
	● Transverse processes (malformation?)
	● Articular processes (shape, no sclerosis, marginal osteophytes)
Interverte-bral disk spaces	● Normal height
Spinal canal	● Normal diameter
Paravertebral lines	● Not widened
	● Not displaced
Ribs	● Shape
	● Position
	● Smooth, intact contours with no discontinuities
Soft tissues	● No foreign bodies or calcifications
	● No swelling

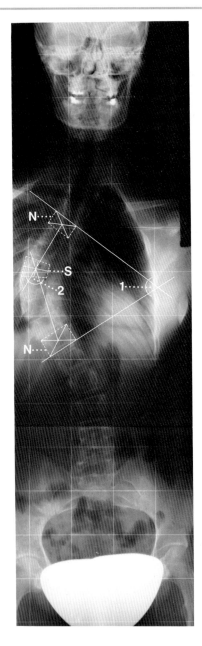

Important Data

Scoliosis angle

1. Cobb measurement: 0° = normal (intersecting perpendiculars to lines through upper and lower end plates)
2. Ferguson measurement: 0° = normal (angle between end vertebra and apical vertebra)

Identifying the *upper and lower end vertebrae* (**N**):

- Rectangular shape
- Maximally tilted from the horizontal
- Minimal rotation (center defined by lines connecting the corners of the vertebral bodies)

  Identifying the *apical vertebra* (**S**):
- Maximal wedging
- (and/or) Maximal rotation (center defined by perpendiculars to the edge bisectors)

Cervical Spine, Biplane Views

The cervical spine shows a physiological degree of lordosis, and the vertebral bodies are normally positioned. The cervical vertebrae are normal in number, shape, and size. The outer contours of the vertebrae, including the end plates, have smooth margins. The uncovertebral joints, apophyseal joints, spinous and transverse processes present a normal shape. The intervertebral disk spaces are of normal height, and the spinal canal is of normal width. The prevertebral fat stripe and the retropharyngeal and retrotracheal spaces are unremarkable.
The trachea and soft tissues show no abnormalities.

Interpretation

The cervical spine appears normal.

Checklist

Position
- Cervical lordosis (no segmental malalignment)
- Variable angle
- Normal frontal and lateral alignment

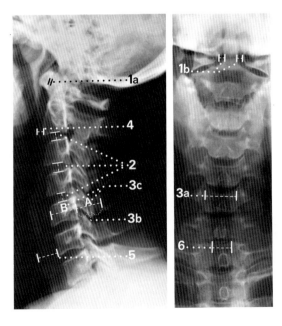

Checklist, continued

Vertebrae number	●	7
Shape	●	Height, size
Structure	●	Mineralization
	●	Normal trabeculation
	●	Sharply defined trabecular pattern
	●	No patchy or linear densities
	●	No lucencies
Contours	●	Cortex, including end plates, is smooth and sharp, with no contour defects
	●	No sclerotic areas or marginal osteophytes
Processes, joints	●	Uncovertebral joints, apophyseal joints (shape, no sclerosis, no wear tracks or marginal osteophytes)
	●	Spinous processes (intact posterior arch)
	●	Transverse processes (shape, smooth and intact contours)
Intervertebral disk spaces	●	Disk height (see below)
	●	No calcifications
Spinal canal	●	Normal sagittal diameter
Paravertebral space	●	Prevertebral fat stripe borders directly on the spine
	●	Retropharyngeal and retrotracheal spaces (see below)
Trachea	●	Centered with normal luminal diameter (see below)
Soft tissues	●	No swelling
	●	No calcifications or foreign bodies

Important Data

1. Atlantoaxial distance:
   (**a**) <3 mm in lateral projection (up to 4 mm in children)
   (**b**) Approximately equal distance in AP projection
2. *Disk height:* C2 < C3 < C4 < C5 < C6 ≥ C7
3. *Width of spinal canal:*
   (**a**) Interpedicular distance (AP projection, C3–C7) = ca. 24–33 mm
   (**b**) Sagittal diameter from vertebral body to vertebral arch = C1 (20–33 mm), C2 (15–29 mm), C3–C7 (ca. 15–24 mm) (FFD [Film-Focus-Distance] = 150 mm); or
   (**c**) Ratio of A:B is greater than 1; or the simple rule:
   (**d**) Vertebral body should fit into the corresponding spinal canal
4. *Width of retropharyngeal space* = 1–7 mm (at C2 level)
5. *Width of retrotracheal space* = 9–22 mm (at C6 level)
6. *Tracheal diameter* = 15–23.5 mm (11.5–18 mm in women)

Cervical Spine, Oblique View

The cervical spine is normally positioned, and the imaged cervical vertebrae are normal in number, shape, structure, and contours. The disk spaces are of proper height. The articular processes and pars interarticularis of each vertebra are normally shaped and have smooth, sharp borders. There is normal separation of the articulating surfaces. The intervertebral foramina have a normal shape and width. Soft-tissue opacities are unremarkable, with no abnormal calcifications or foreign bodies.

Interpretation

The intervertebral foramina of the cervical spine appear normal, with no evidence of anterior or posterior narrowing.

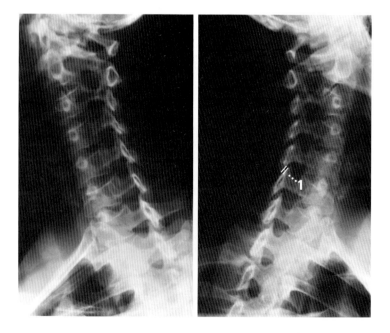

Checklist

Position	●	Harmonious axis
	●	Normal vertebral alignment
	●	No displacement of individual vertebral bodies
Vertebrae number	●	7
Shape	●	Scalloped rectangle (C3–C7 vertebral bodies)
Structure	●	Mineralization
	●	Normal arrangement of cancellous trabeculae
	●	Sharply defined trabecular pattern
	●	No patchy densities
	●	No lucencies
Contours	●	Cortex is smooth and sharp
	●	No contour defects
	●	No sclerosis
	●	No marginal osteophytes
Intervertebral disk spaces	●	Normal height (compared with adjacent disk spaces)
Apophyseal joints	●	Shape
	●	Position
	●	Articulating surfaces (smooth, sharp margins, no spurs or increased sclerosis)
	●	Width of joint space (see below)
Pars inter-articularis	●	Shape
	●	Intact contours
	●	No slitlike lucent lines
Intervertebral foramina	●	Elliptical shape
	●	No encroachment from the anterior side (uncinate process) or posterior side (spondylarthrosis)
	●	No widening (compared with adjacent foramina)
Soft tissues	●	No calcifications or foreign bodies

Important Data

1. Width of apophyseal joint spaces = 1.5–2 mm

Cervical Spine, Functional Views

Lateral projections demonstrate a normal position of the cervical spine in maximal flexion and extension. The posterior margins of the verte-

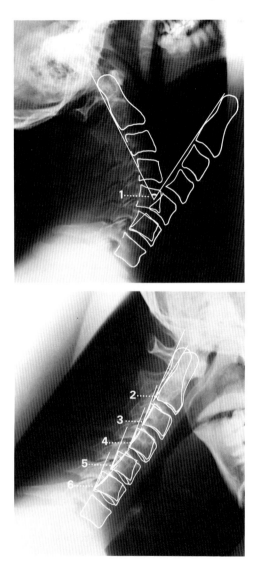

bral bodies in flexion show a physiological stair-step configuration. There is no pathological anterior or posterior displacement of individual vertebral bodies. All of the disk spaces present a normal shape on flexion views. The ranges of flexion and extension as determined from the motion diagram are normal from C2 to C7.

Interpretation

The cervical spine shows a normal range of flexion–extension with no segmental abnormalities.

Checklist

Position (cervical spine)	• Normal maximal flexion–extension (see below) (extension views are contraindicated in fresh trauma cases!)
	• Coordinated function of the atlas and axis
Position (of individual vertebral bodies)	• Physiological stair-step configuration of vertebral-body posterior margins in flexion view
	• No pathological anterior or posterior displacement (slippage, drawer phenomenon)
	• No fixed axial malalignment (stepoff)
	• Disk spaces: uniform wedge shape
	• No segmental restriction
Motion diagram	• Normal (see below)

Important Data

1. Range of maximal flexion–extension in the cervical spine: from 19° to 54°

Angles in motion diagram:

2. C2–C3: 5–18°
3. C3–C4: 12–23°
4. C4–C5: 16–28°
5. C5–C6: 18–28°
6. C6–C7: 13–25°

Thoracic Spine, Biplane Views

The lateral projection shows harmonious, physiological kyphosis of the thoracic spine. The thoracic vertebrae are normal in number, shape, size, and interrelationships, with proper mineralization and bone structure. The cortical margins, including the end plates, are smooth and sharply defined. The pedicles and the spinous, transverse, and articular processes show a normal configuration. The costotransverse and costovertebral joints have a normal shape.

The disk spaces are of normal height, and the spinal canal is of normal width. Imaged portions of the ribs are unremarkable.

The imaged soft tissues contain no radiopaque foreign bodies.

Interpretation

The thoracic spine appears normal.

Checklist

Position	• Axis (physiological kyphosis, see below)
	• Normal vertebral alignment
	• No segmental malalignment
Vertebrae number	• 12
Shape	• Rectangular (see below)
Structure	• Mineralization
	• Normal trabeculation
	• No patchy or linear densities
	• No lucencies
Contours	• Cortex, including end plates, is smooth and sharp
	• No contour defects (impressions)
	• No sclerosis
	• No marginal osteophytes
Posterior elements	• Spinous processes (shape, smooth and intact contours, no contact between adjacent processes)
	• Transverse processes (shape, costotransverse joints: no marginal osteophytes or sclerosis)
	• Articular processes (shape, smooth articular surfaces, no sclerosis or marginal osteophytes)
Disk spaces	• Normal height (see below)
	• No vacuum phenomenon
	• No disk calcifications
Spinal canal	• Normal width (see below)
Paravertebral lines	• Not widened (see below)
	• Not displaced
Ribs	• Shape, position
	• Smooth, intact contours with no discontinuities
	• No densities or lucencies
	• No ulcerations
Soft tissues	• No foreign bodies or calcifications
	• No soft-tissue masses

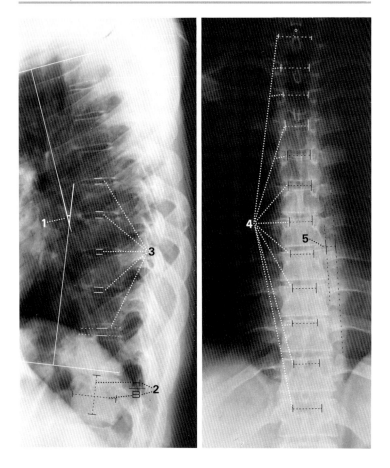

Important Data

1. *Kyphosis angle* measured by the Stagnara technique:
   Angle between the end plates of T3 and T11 = 25 °
2. *Shape* (T12): height/width = 0.83 (0.93 in women)
3. *Height of disk spaces:*
   T6–T11: ca. 4–5 mm
   T11–T12: ca. 6.5 mm
   Lowest at T1
4. *Width of spinal canal:*
   Interpedicular distance (AP projection): T1 (20–27 mm) > T2 >
   T3 >T4 > T5 = T6 (15–20 mm) = T7, T8 < T9 < T10 < T11 < T12
   (19–27 mm)
5. *Paravertebral lines:* under age 40 years = 6–8 mm; over age 40
   years = 6–15 mm
   (Usually visible only on the left side from T4 to T11)

Lumbar Spine, Biplane Views

The lateral projection shows harmonious, physiological lordosis of the lumbar spine. The lumbar vertebrae are normal in number, shape, size, and interrelationships, with proper mineralization and bone structure. The cortical borders, including the end plates, are smoothly marginated. The pedicles and the spinous, transverse and articular processes show a normal configuration. The disk spaces are of normal height, and the spinal canal is of normal width.

The imaged soft tissues contain no foreign bodies or calcifications.

Interpretation

The lumbar spine appears normal.

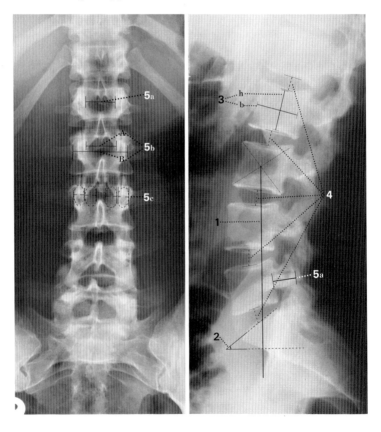

Checklist

Position	• Lumbar lordosis, static axis (see below)
	• Normal vertebral alignment
	• No segmental malalignment
Number of vertebrae	• 5 (L3 has the largest transverse processes; the transverse processes of L4 point cephalad)
Shape	• Scalloped rectangle (see below)
Structure	• Mineralization
	• Normal trabeculation
	• Sharply defined trabecular pattern
	• No patchy or linear densities
	• No lucencies
Contours	• Cortex, including the end plates, is smooth and sharp
	• No contour defects
	• No sclerosis
	• No marginal osteophytes
Pedicles	• Elliptical, paired, symmetrical
Processes	• Spinous processes (shape, smooth and intact contours, no contact between adjacent processes)
	• Transverse processes (shape, no contour defects)
	• Articular processes (shape, smooth articular surfaces, no increased sclerosis or marginal osteophytes)
Disk spaces	• Normal height (see below)
	• No vacuum phenomenon, no disk calcifications
Spinal canal	• Normal width (see below)
Soft tissues	• No foreign bodies or calcifications
	• Sharp delineation of psoas margins

Important Data

1. *Static axis:* plumb line from center of L3 intersects S1
2. *Lumbosacral angle* (S1/horizonal plane) = 26–57° (ca. 34°)
3. *Shape:* height/width (L1–L3) = 0.87 (1.0 in women)
4. *Height of disk spaces:* L1 < L2 < L3 < L4 > L5
5. *Width of spinal canal:*
   (**a**) Interpedicular distance (AP projection): greater than 16 mm
   Sagittal diameter: greater than 11; or
   (**b**) A:B < 0.5 = suspicious for spinal stenosis; or the following simple rule:
   (**c**) If the spinal canal diameter is normal, both pedicles should fit side-by-side into the space between them. If they do not fit, the spinal canal is too narrow. If more than two would fit, the spinal canal is too wide (mass?)

Lumbar Spine, Oblique View

The position of the lumbar spine is normal, and the lumbar vertebrae are normal in their number, shape, structure, and contours. The disk spaces are of proper height.

The pars interarticularis and posterior arch of each vertebra appear normal, and there are no demonstrable pars or arch defects. The articular processes present a normal shape. The articulating surfaces are smooth and sharply defined and show a normal degree of separation.

The soft tissues are unremarkable.

Interpretation

No pars abnormalities are observed in the lumbar vertebrae.

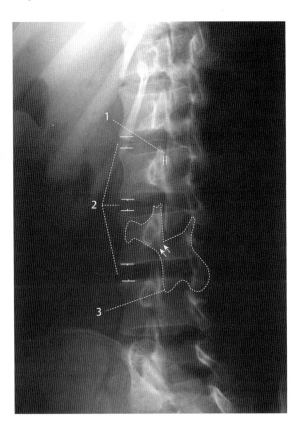

Checklist

Position	• Physiological lordosis
	• Normal vertebral alignment
Vertebrae number	• 5
Shape	• Scalloped rectangular shape
Structure	• Mineralization
	• Normal trabeculation
	• Sharply defined trabecular pattern
	• No abnormal densities or lucencies
Contours	• Cortex is smooth and sharp
	• No contour defects
	• No sclerosis or marginal osteophytes
Disk spaces	• Normal height (see below)
	• No calcifications
	• No vacuum phenomenon
Pars inter-articularis	• Shape
	• No lengthening or narrowing of pars isthmus
	• Contours (intact)
	• Lachapel's "collarless dog" figure (see below)
	• No cleftlike lucent lines or defects
Apophyseal joints	• Shape
	• Position
	• Articulating surfaces (smooth, sharp margins)
	• No marginal osteophytes
	• No increased sclerosis
	• Width of joint space (see below)
Soft tissues	• No calcifications or foreign bodies

Important Data

1. *Width of apophyseal joint spaces:* 1.5–2 mm
2. *Height of disk spaces:* L1/L2 < L2/L3 < L4/L5 > L5/S1 (usually difficult to evaluate in oblique views)
3. "Collarless dog" figure (arrows) confirms absence of pars defect

Lumbar Spine, Functional Views

Lateral views in maximal flexion and extension demonstrate normal functional curvatures of the lumbar spine. The individual vertebral bodies show no pathological anterior or posterior displacements. The disk spaces show a consistent, physiological shape (anterior taper) in the flexion views. The motion diagram is normal.

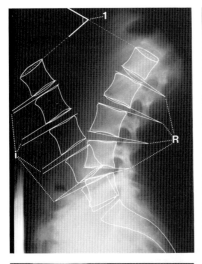

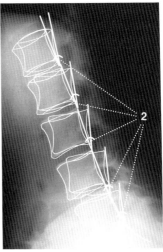

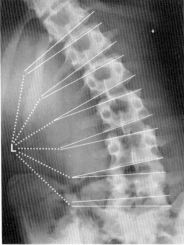

Interpretation

The lumbar spine displays normal flexion and extension.

Checklist

Axis
- Smooth alignment curves (e.g., of the spinous processes on sidebending)

Lumbar spine
- No segmental malalignment

Position of individual vertebral bodies
- Interrelationship of the vertebral bodies (no anterior or posterior displacement)
- No hypermobility or hypomobility compared with surrounding disk spaces
- No fixed axial malalignment (stepoff)
- No drawer phenomenon
- No abnormal straightening of several vertebrae above a loose segment (Güntz's sign)

Disk spaces
- On lumbar flexion, the anterior margins of the vertebral bodies move closer together while the disk spaces taper anteriorly (i)
- On lumbar extension, the disk spaces taper posteriorly (R)
- On sidebending, the margins of the vertebral bodies move closer together on the concave side while the disk spaces taper laterally (L)
- Important: Watch for absence of disk-space wedging in just one or two segments, especially if wedging is preserved on sidebending to the opposite side

---

Important Data

1. Total range of motion of the lumbar spine = approx. 64° (to 80°) (Bakke measurement)
2. Mobility of individual vertebral bodies during maximal flexion–extension = 8–18° (Burri measurement)

   Mobility usually increases from L1/L2 to L4/L5 and is usually maximal at L4/L5

   Mobility is highly variable at L5/S1, but this segment is the least mobile on lateral bending

Pelvis, Standing Anteroposterior View

The pelvic skeleton presents an anatomically normal and symmetrical shape. The superior borders of the iliac wings are at equal levels. The bone displays proper structure and mineralization. The cortical borders are of normal thickness, smooth, and sharply defined with no pathological contour defects. The acetabular roof appears normal on each side.

The femoral heads are normal in shape and position. The articular surfaces are smooth and sharply defined, congruent, and are separated by a joint space of normal width. There are no intra-articular or periarticular calcifications.

The sacroiliac joint and symphysis pubis are of normal width and have smooth, sharp borders. The sacrum and imaged portions of the lumbar spine are unremarkable.

The soft tissues contain no abnormal calcifications or radiopaque foreign bodies.

Interpretation

The pelvis appears normal.

Checklist

Shape	•	Symmetrical
Position	•	Superior pelvic margins are at equal levels (only on standing radiograph)
Structure	•	Mineralization
	•	Sharply defined trabecular pattern
	•	No circumscribed lucencies or densities
Contours	•	Smooth, sharp cortex
	•	Normal cortical bone thickness (compared with opposite side)
	•	No contour defects or discontinuities
	•	No bony excrescences (especially on the ischia or the anterior superior or inferior iliac spine)
	•	No subperiosteal sclerosis or elevation
Hip	•	Acetabular roof:
		— Shape (symmetry)
		— Köhler teardrop figure
	•	Femoral head:
		— Shape

Checklist, continued

- — CCD angle (see below)
- — Position (projection should demonstrate greater and lesser trochanters!)
- • Hip joint:
  - — Articular surfaces (smooth, sharp)
  - — Joint space (see below)
  - — No marginal osteophytes (acetabular roof, femoral head, fovea)
  - — No subchondral sclerosis or subcortical cystic lucencies
  - — No intra-articular or periarticular calcifications

Symphysis pubis
- • Width of symphysis (see below)
- • No marginal osteophytes
- • No subchondral sclerosis, cysts, or erosions

Sacroiliac joint
- • Shape of joint
- • Contours (smooth, sharp)
- • Width of joint space (see below)
- • No local expansions or sclerosis
- • No subcortical lucencies or densities
- • No cysts

Sacrum
- • Structure
- • Contours and foraminal outlines are smooth and sharp (equal on both sides?)

Lumbar spine
- • Axis (straight)
- • Shape of vertebral bodies
- • Bone structure
- • Contours (marginal osteophytes?)
- • Pedicles intact

Soft tissues
- • No soft-tissue density or swelling
- • No radiopaque foreign bodies
- • No calcifications (vascular or at tendon attachments)
- • Fat pad (hip) not elevated
- • Urinary bladder
- • Line of obturator internus muscle (hematoma, coxarthritis)
- • If evaluable: lines of the piriformis, psoas margin, levator ani

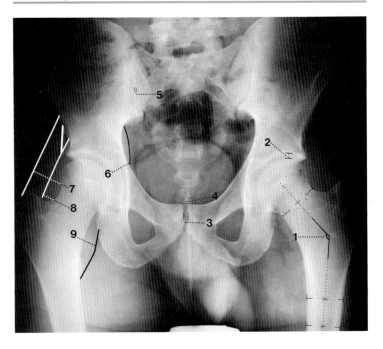

Important Data

1. *CCD angle:* 120–130°
2. *Width of joint space:* 4–5 mm
3. *Width of symphysis:* up to 6 mm (multipara)
4. *Unilateral elevation of symphysis:* maximum of 2 mm
5. Width of *sacroiliac joint space:* 3–4 mm
6. *Soft-tissue line:* obturator internus
7. *Fat stripe* between gluteus minimus and medius
8. *Fat stripe* medial to gluteus minimus
9. *Fat stripe* medial to iliopsoas

Pelvis, Martius View

The pelvic skeleton presents an anatomically normal and symmetrical shape, with a normal position of the imaged skeletal structures. The pelvic inlet has a physiological configuration and smooth boundaries. Measurements of the true conjugate, oblique diameter, and transverse diameter are within normal limits.

The rest of the pelvic skeleton appears normal.

The soft tissues are unremarkable.

Interpretation

The pelvic skeleton and pelvic inlet appear normal.

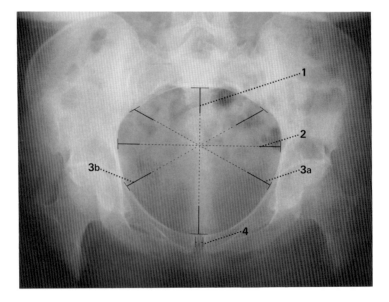

Checklist

Shape	• Iliac wings (symmetry)
	• Sacrum and lumbar spine
	• Transverse elliptical shape of the pelvic inlet (an accurate projection should superimpose the pubic and ischial rami)
Position	• Superior pelvic margins are approximately at equal levels
	• Sacrum and coccyx are on the midline
Pelvic inlet	• Inner margin of the pelvic ring (pubis, iliac wings, sacrum, promontory) has smooth, even contours
	• No discontinuities
	• No bony excrescences
	• Normal width of symphysis pubis (see below), no stepoff
	• Normal dimensions:
	1. True (obstetric) conjugate (see below)
	2. Transverse diameter (see below)
	3. Oblique diameter (see below)
	(1st oblique diameter: from left iliopubic eminence to contralateral sacroiliac joint; 2nd oblique diameter: from right eminence to left sacroiliac joint)
Other skeletal structures	• Bone structure
	• Contours
	• Position of hip and lower lumbar spine
	• Sacroiliac joint (shape, width, borders)
Soft tissues	• No calcifications (especially intrapelvic)
	• No foreign bodies
	• No soft-tissue swelling
	• Distribution of bowel gas

Important Data

1. *True (obstetric) conjugate* = ca. 11 cm
2. *Transverse diameter* = ca. 13 cm
3. *Oblique diameter* = approx. 12 cm
   (**a**) First oblique diameter
   (**b**) Second oblique diameter
4. *Width of symphysis:* up to 6 mm (multipara)

Pelvis, Guthmann View

The lumbar spine, sacrum, and coccyx show normal relative positions. The bony boundaries of the pelvic cavity have a normal configuration and smooth contours. Measurements of the true conjugate, pelvic cavity, and longitudinal diameter of the pelvic outlet are within normal limits.

Other skeletal structures appear normal.

The soft tissues are unremarkable.

Interpretation

The lateral pelvis appears normal, and pelvic dimensions are within normal limits.

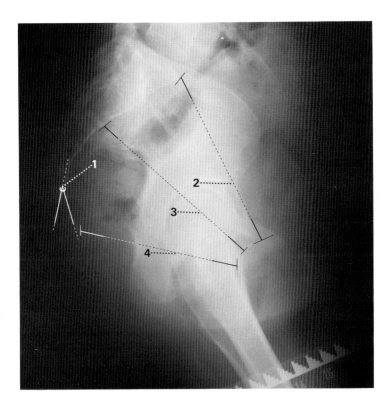

Checklist

Shape	• Accurate projection (superimposing the femoral heads)
	• Normal lumbosacral angle
	• Relation of L5 to the sacrum
	• Relation of the coccyx to the sacrum (see below)
Pelvic inlet	• True (obstetric) conjugate (see below)
	• Normal lumbosacral junction
	• No bony excrescences
Pelvic cavity	• Normal curvature of the anterior surfaces of the sacrum and coccyx
	• Dimensions (see below)
Pelvic outlet	• Longitudinal diameter (see below)
Rest of skeleton	• Lower lumbar spine, sacrum, coccyx:
	— Shape, position, structure, contours, disk spaces
	— Gross abnormalities of the articular surfaces
Soft tissues	• No calcifications (especially intrapelvic)
	• No foreign bodies
	• No soft-tissue swelling

Important Data

1. Anterior angle between coccyx and sacrum = ca. 10–30° (highly variable)
2. *Pelvic inlet (true conjugate)* = ca. 11 cm
3. *Pelvic cavity:* greater than 12 cm
4. *Pelvic outlet:* ca. 9 cm

Iliac Wing and Obturator Views

The acetabulum has a normal shape, and its margins and floor appear normal. The cortical margins are smooth and sharply defined. There is no sign of pathological contour defects or abnormal lucencies or densities. There are no marginal osteophytes.

The joint space is of normal width. The articular surfaces are congruent, and the femoral head is smoothly outlined and well covered by the acetabular roof. The pubis and ischium are normally shaped.

The obturator foramen is well defined. Its cortical margins are intact, and its bone structure is unremarkable. The iliac wing is normal in its shape, outlines, and bone structure.

The soft tissues are unremarkable.

Interpretation

The hip joint appears normal. In particular, there are no abnormalities involving the acetabulum, the acetabular pillars, the pubis, ischium, or iliac wing.

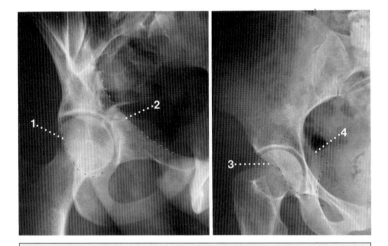

Important Data

Bone lines:
1. Posterior acetablular margin   3. Anterior acetabular margin
2. Linea terminalis (pelvic inlet) 4. Ischium

Checklist

Acetabulum	• Anterior acetabular margin, best appreciated in the iliac wing view (right image)
	• Posterior acetabular margin, best appreciated in the obturator view (left image)
	• Floor of acetabulum
Joint, femoral head	• Medial joint space and femoral head (obturator)
	• Anterior and posterior joint space, femoral head (iliac wing)
Pubis, ischium	• Obturator view—useful for evaluating:

  − Linea terminalis

  − Medial and lower part of ischium

  − Obturator foramen (elliptical shape)

  − Ischium

 • Iliac wing view—useful for evaluating:

  − Lateral part of ischium

  − Ischial spine

  − Pubis

Iliac wing

Shape • Best appreciated on the iliac wing view

 • Note particularly the femoral head, acetabulum (congruity of articular surfaces, femoral head coverage), and iliac wing

Structure

 • Mineralization

 • Normal arrangement of cancellous trabeculae

 • Sharply defined trabecular pattern

 • No abnormal lucencies or densities

Contours

 • Cortex smooth and sharp

 • Normal cortical bone thickness

 • No contour defects or discontinuities

 • No marginal osteophytes (acetabular roof, femoral head, fovea)

 • No bony excrescences (especially on the ischia or the anterior superior or inferior iliac spine)

 • No subperiosteal sclerosis or elevation

Soft tissues

 • No soft-tissue density or swelling

 • No radiopaque foreign bodies

 • No calcifications (intra-articular or periarticular, vascular, or at tendon attachments)

 • Fat pad (hip) not elevated

 • Urinary bladder

 • Line of obturator internus (hematoma, coxarthritis)

Sacroiliac Joint, Anteroposterior View

The articular surfaces of the sacroiliac joint are normally shaped. Their cortical borders are smooth, sharp, and of proper thickness with no abnormal contour defects. The joint space is of normal width.
Imaged portions of the ilium and sacrum are normally shaped and symmetrical, with proper mineralization and bone structure.
The soft tissues are unremarkable, with no signs of calcifications or radiopaque foreign bodies.

Interpretation

The sacroiliac joints appear normal

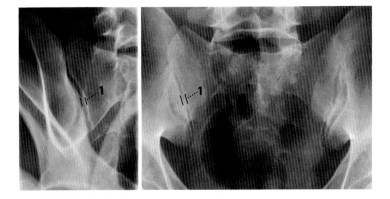

Checklist

Joint	● Articular surfaces are convergent inferiorly (and symmetrical)
Shape	● Two views are available:
	— AP projection with the lumbar spine straightened
	— AP projection with the ipsilateral side elevated ca. 30°
Contours	● Cortex smooth and sharp, normal cortical bone thickness
	● No contour defects or discontinuities
	● No bandlike, patchy, or circumscribed densities
	● No erosion, destruction, or cysts
	● No sclerosis
	● No marginal osteophytes
Joint	● Normal width of joint space (see below)
	● No circumscribed widening
	● No ankylosis
	● No lucencies (air)
Bone	
Shape	● Sacrum (4 pairs of foramina, 5 vertebrae): symmetrical
Structure	● Mineralization
	● Sharp delineation of cancellous trabecular structure (including subchondral articular bone)
	● No circumscribed densities or lucencies
Soft tissues	● No calcification of tendons or fasciae
	● No radiopaque foreign bodies or calcifications (lymph nodes, vessels)

Important Data

1. Width of sacroiliac joint space = 3–4 mm

Sacrum, Biplane Views

The sacrum and coccyx have an anatomically normal shape, with symmetrical inferior tapering of the coccygeal vertebrae. The coccyx occupies a normal position with no significant lateral or anterior angulation. The sacrum and coccyx show proper mineralization and bone structure. The articular surfaces of the sacroiliac joint present a normal shape, contours, and joint space. The foraminal boundaries and the contours of the coccygeal vertebrae are smooth and sharp with no contour defects. The soft tissues are unremarkable.

Interpretation

The sacrum and coccyx appear normal.

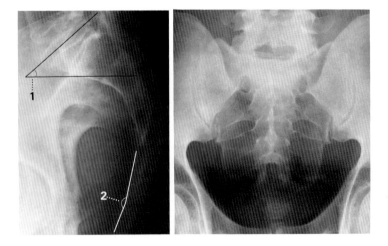

Checklist

Shape	• Sacrum:
	– 4 pairs of foramina (5 vertebrae)
	– Symmetry
	– Harmonious curvature of the sacral anterior surface (lateral projection)
	• Coccyx:
	– Triangular shape (if evaluable)
	– Number (4 or 5 rudimentary vertebrae)
	– Size (no atypical shortening or elongation)
	– No broadening or deformity
	– Symmetrical inferior taper
Position	• Lumbosacral angle (see below)
	• Relation of L5 to sacrum
	• Relation of coccyx to sacrum (see below)
	• No angulation of the coccyx (especially anterior)
Structure	• Mineralization
	• No circumscribed densities
	• No lucencies or expansions
Contours	• Cortex (smooth, sharp, normal thickness)
	• No contour defects or discontinuities
	• *Sacroiliac joint and disk spaces:*
	– Smooth articular surfaces
	– Normal cortical bone thickness
	– No sclerosis
	– No marginal osteophytes
	– No lucencies or densities
	– Normal width of joint space (if evaluable)
	• *Foraminal boundaries:*
	– Smooth and sharp
	– No contour defects or discontinuities
Soft tissues	• Calcifications, foreign bodies?

Important Data

1. Lumbosacral angle (S1/horizontal plane) = 26–57° (ca. 34°) (horizontal plane is perpendicular to a line connecting the symphysis with the anterior superior iliac spine)
2. Relation of coccyx to sacrum: anterior angle of approx. 10–30° (in lateral projection, highly variable)

Coccyx, Biplane Views

The coccyx has a normal shape, with symmetrical inferior tapering of the coccygeal vertebrae. The axial alignment of the coccyx is anatomically normal with no significant lateral or anterior angulation. The vertebrae show proper mineralization and bone structure. The outlines of the vertebral bodies are smooth and sharply defined with no contour defects.

Imaged portions of the sacrum are unremarkable.

The soft tissues are normal.

Interpretation

The coccyx appears normal.

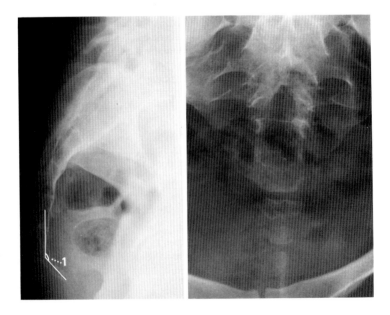

Checklist

Shape	●	Triangular
	●	Normal number of vertebral bodies (see below)
	●	Normal size (no atypical shortening or elongation)
	●	No broadening or deformity
	●	Symmetrical inferior taper
Position	●	Normal axial alignment (see below)
	●	No angulation (anterior)
Structure	●	Mineralization
	●	No circumscribed densities
	●	No lucencies or expansions
Contours	●	Cortex (smooth, sharp)
	●	No contour defects
Sacrum	●	Shape
	●	Position
	●	Bone structure
	●	Sacroiliac joints
Soft tissues	●	No calcifications
	●	No foreign bodies

Important Data

Coccyx is comprised of 3 or 4 vertebral bodies
1. Relation to sacrum: anterior angle of approx. 10°–30° (in lateral projection, highly variable)

The Upper Extremity

Bony Hemithorax

The ribs are normal in shape, number, and position. The intercostal spaces are of normal width.

Mineralization and bone structure are normal. The cortex has smooth, sharp margins with no pathological contour defects. Cortical bone thickness is normal. The costovertebral and costotransverse joints have an anatomically normal shape.

No abnormalities are visible in the soft tissues or in imaged portions of the lung, heart, and mediastinum.

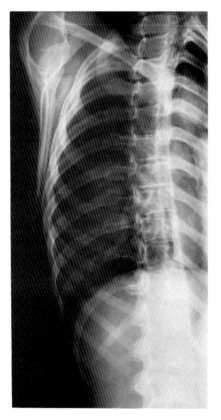

Interpretation

The bony hemithorax appears normal.

Checklist

Shape	• Number (12 pairs of ribs)
	• Rib shape (bifurcated, fused?)
	• Thoracic shape
Position	• Parallel arrangement of the ribs
	• Posterior part is horizontal, anterior part is directed inferiorly
	• Uniform width of intercostal spaces
Structure	• Mineralization
	• Normal trabeculation
	• Sharp delineation of the trabecular pattern
	• No circumscribed lucencies or densities
	• No expansions
	• Moderate calcification of the costal cartilages, corresponding to the course of the ribs
Contours	• Cortex smooth and sharp
	• Normal cortical bone thickness
	• No contour defects or discontinuities
	• No periosteal reaction or elevation
	• No sclerosis
	• No erosions or ulcerations (especially in inferior rib margins)
Joints	• Costovertebral and costotransverse joints:
	– Smooth, sharp margins of joint space
	– No marginal osteophytes or sclerosis
Soft tissues	• No soft-tissue swelling (cutaneous emphysema?)
	• No pleural thickening
	• No gross abnormalities of pulmonary structure
	• Heart (enlargement, calcium)
	• Mediastinum (position, shape, abnormal shadowing or lucency, trachea)
	• No radiopaque foreign bodies or calcifications

Sternum, Biplane Views

The sternum shows an anatomically normal shape, position, and curvature. Its mineralization and bone structure are normal. Its cortical margins are smooth and sharp with no contour defects. The visible portions of both clavicles have a normal shape and position. The articulating surfaces of the sternoclavicular joint have smooth, sharp borders and a joint space of normal width. The pleural surface of the sternum appears normal.

The soft-tissue envelope is unremarkable.

Interpretation

The sternum and sternoclavicular joints appear normal.

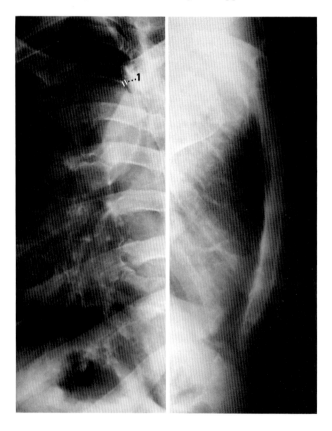

Checklist

Shape (position)	• Normal curvature
	• No abnormal sternal prominence or depression (pectus deformity)
	• Configuration of the xiphoid (no significant anterior or posterior curvature)
Structure	• Mineralization
	• No circumscribed lucencies or densities
Contours	• Cortical bone smooth and sharp
	• Normal cortical bone thickness (no circumscribed thickening or thinning)
	• No contour defects or discontinuities
	• Superior sternal synchondrosis smooth and sharply defined (no contour defects, marginal osteophytes, or fusion)
Joints	• Clavicles (shape, relation to manubrium sterni)
	• Articular surfaces (smooth, sharp)
	• No sclerosis
	• No marginal osteophytes
	• No ulcerations
	• Width of joint space (see below) (equal on both sides)
	• No intra-articular or periarticular calcifications
Soft tissues	• No widening of anterior pleural contact line
	• Normal thickness of chest wall
	• No calcifications or foreign bodies

Important Data

1. Width of sternoclavicular joint space = 3–5 mm

Anteroposterior Weight-Bearing View of the Shoulders

The bones comprising the shoulder joints have a normal, symmetrical shape. The acromion and clavicle are at approximately equal levels on both sides, and their joint spaces are of proper width. The humeral heads show normal, symmetrical articulation on both sides. The sterno-clavicular joints are normal and symmetrical.

Imaged portions of the upper ribs are normal in shape and number. The lower cervical spine and upper thoracic spine are normally positioned and show proper mineralization and bone structure. The outlines of the bones and articular surfaces are smooth and sharply defined. There are no intra-articular or periarticular calcifications.

The soft tissues are unremarkable.

Interpretation

Both shoulder joints appear normal and symmetrical.

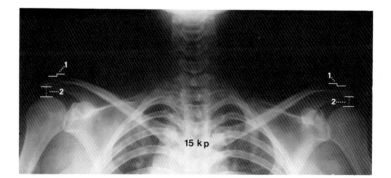

Checklist

Shape	• Clavicles (symmetrical, no angulation)
	• Scapulae (symmetrical)
	• Humeral heads (rounded, symmetrical)
	• Ribs (prominence of visible segments, no super-numerary ribs, cervical ribs)
	• Cervical spine
Position	• Acromioclavicular joints are at approximately equal levels on both sides, with no right–left discrepancy (with both arms carrying a weight of 15 kg each)
	• Scapulae have the same position on both sides
	• Normal position of the ribs and cervical spine
	• Symmetrical articulation in the sternoclavicular joint
Structure	• Mineralization
	• Normal trabeculation
	• Sharp delineation of the trabecular pattern (if evaluable)
	• No circumscribed lucencies or densities
	• Epiphyseal plates (open/closed)
Contours	• Cortex smooth and sharp
	• No circumscribed thickening or thinning (compared with opposite side)
	• No contour defects or discontinuities
	• No marginal osteophytes
Soft tissues	• Intact
	• No swelling
	• No foreign bodies
	• Fat pad apposed to the bone (especially near the joint)
	• No calcifications (vascular, intra-articular or peri-articular)

Important Data

1. Acromioclavicular joints are at approximately the same level on both sides
2. Humeral heads are at approximately the same level on both sides

Clavicle

The clavicle shows an anatomically normal shape and position with proper mineralization and bone structure. The cortical bone has smooth, sharp contours and normal thickness with no pathological contour defects.

The articular surfaces of the acromioclavicular and sternoclavicular joints are smooth and sharply defined. The joint spaces are of normal width.

Visible portions of the ribs, scapula, and humerus are unremarkable. The soft tissues show no abnormalities.

Interpretation

The clavicle appears normal.

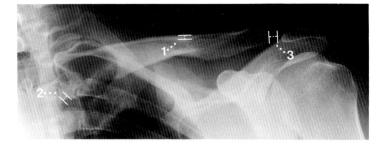

Checklist

Shape	•	Long tubular bone
	•	No angulation
Position	•	Compare proximal end of clavicle at manubrium sterni with the opposite side
	•	Distal end is level with the acromion
Structure	•	Mineralization
	•	Normal trabeculation
	•	Sharp delineation of the trabecular pattern
	•	No circumscribed lucencies, expansions, or densities
	•	Normal width of medullary canals
	•	Epiphyseal plates (open/closed)
Contours	•	Cortex smooth and sharp
	•	Normal cortical bone thickness (see below)
	•	No contour defects or discontinuities
	•	No periosteal reaction or elevation
Joints	•	Acromioclavicular and sternoclavicular joints:
		— Shape
		— Contours (smooth, sharp)
		— No sclerosis, no subchondral lucencies
		— Width of joint space (see below)
		— No (intra-articular or) periarticular calcifications
Other bones	•	Ribs, scapula, humerus:
		— Shape
		— Position
		— Structure
		— Contours
Soft tissues	•	Intact
	•	No swelling
	•	No foreign bodies
	•	Fat pad apposed to the bone (especially near the joint)
	•	No calcifications (vascular or at tendon attachments)

Important Data

1. Cortical bone thickness = 2–4 mm
2. Width of sternoclavicular joint space = 3–5 mm
3. Width of acromioclavicular joint space = 2–4 mm

Acromioclavicular Joint

Imaged skeletal structures have an anatomically normal shape. The acromion and clavicle show a normal position and interrelationship. Mineralization and bone structure are normal.

The cortex is intact and has smooth, sharp margins. Cortical bone thickness is normal.

The articular surfaces present normal contours. The joint space is of normal width.

The soft tissues are unremarkable.

Interpretation

The acromioclavicular joint appears normal.

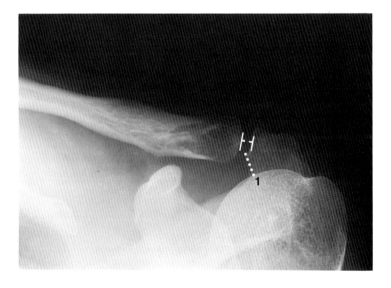

Checklist

Shape	• Acromion
	• End of clavicle
	• Coracoid (humeral head)
Position	• Clavicle and acromion are at approximately the same level
	• Position of the humeral head (if evaluable)
Structure	• Mineralization
	• Normal trabeculation
	• Sharp delineation of the trabecular pattern
	• No circumscribed lucencies or densities
	• Epiphyseal plates (open/closed)
Contours	• Cortex smooth and sharp
	• Normal cortical bone thickness (see below)
	• No contour defects or discontinuities
	• No marginal osteophytes or sclerotic areas
	• Intact subchondral plate
	• No erosions
	• No subperiosteal bone resorption (especially at the inferior clavicular border)
	• Width of joint space (see below)
Soft tissues	• Intact
	• No swelling
	• No foreign bodies
	• No calcifications (vascular, intra-articular or periarticular, at tendon attachments)

Important Data

1. Width of acromioclavicular joint space = 2–4 mm

Scapula, Biplane Views

The scapula has an anatomically normal shape with proper mineralization and bone structure. The bony contours are smooth and sharply defined.

The shoulder joint and acromioclavicular joint have smooth articular surfaces and a normal appearance.

Imaged portions of the humeral head, clavicle, and ribs are normally positioned and unremarkable. There are no intra-articular or periarticular calcifications.

The soft tissues are normal.

Interpretation

The scapula appears normal.

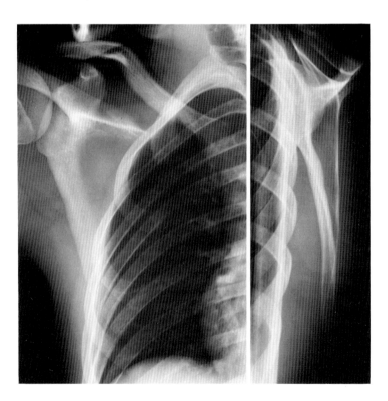

Checklist

Shape	• Scapula (triangular), coracoid, acromion (articular surface) and, if visible, the clavicle and humeral head (spherical)
Position	• Scapula: between the 2nd and 8th ribs
Structure	• Mineralization
	• Normal trabeculation
	• Sharp delineation of trabecular pattern
	• No circumscribed lucencies or densities (progressive decalcification is normal with aging; compare equivocal findings with the opposite side)
	• No fracture lines
Contours	• Cortex smooth and sharp
	• No contour defects or discontinuities
	• No marginal osteophytes
	• No exostoses (especially at the superior angle)
Joints	• *Shoulder joint:*
	— Shape
	— Position
	— Smooth, intact contours
	— No marginal osteophytes
	— No sclerotic areas
	— Normal width of joint space
	— Normal bone structure of humeral head
	• *Acromioclavicular joint:*
	— Shape
	— Position (acromion and clavicle at approximately the same level)
	— Width of joint space
	— Smooth, intact contours
	— No erosions
Soft tissues	• Intact
	• No swelling
	• No foreign bodies
	• No calcifications (vascular, intra-articular or periarticular, at tendon attachments)

Shoulder Joint, Biplane Views

The bones comprising the shoulder joint present a normal shape, with normal articulation of the humeral head. Mineralization and bone structure are normal. The articular surfaces have normal contours. The joint space is of normal width throughout.

Other adjacent bones of the shoulder girdle and upper thoracic skeleton are unremarkable.

The soft tissues are normal.

Interpretation

The shoulder joint appears normal.

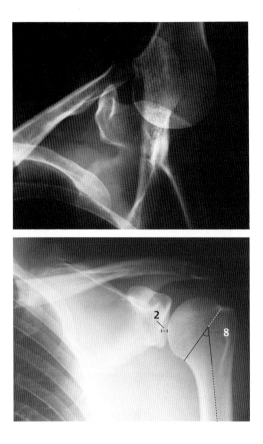

Checklist

Shape	• Spherical humeral head
	• Glenoid, humerus, scapula
Position	• Articulation of humeral head
	• Angle (see below)
Structure	• Mineralization
	• Normal trabeculation
	• Sharp delineation of trabecular pattern
	• No circumscribed lucencies or densities (especially in the lateral part of the humeral head)
	• Epiphyseal plates (open/closed)
Joint	• Contours: cortex smooth and sharp
	• No circumscribed thickening or thinning
	• No contour defects or discontinuities
	• No marginal osteophytes or sclerosis
	• Width of joint space (see below)
	• No intra- or periarticular calcifications
Other bones	• Contours: cortex smooth and sharp
	• Normal cortical bone thickness
	• No contour defects or discontinuities
	• No periosteal reaction or elevation
Soft tissues	• Intact
	• No swelling
	• No foreign bodies
	• Fat pad apposed to the bone (especially near the joint)
	• No calcifications (vascular, intra-articular or peri-articular, at tendon attachments)

Important Data

1. Angle between humeral axis and anatomical neck of humerus = 60–62°
2. Width of joint space = 4–6 mm

Axial Shoulder View

The humeral head, glenoid, and other bones comprising the shoulder joint present a normal shape. The humeral head shows normal articulation.

Mineralization and bone structure are normal.

The cortical margins of the articular surfaces are smooth and intact, and the joint space is of proper width. The other bones comprising the shoulder joint are unremarkable.

The imaged soft tissues show no abnormalities.

Interpretation

The shoulder joint appears normal.

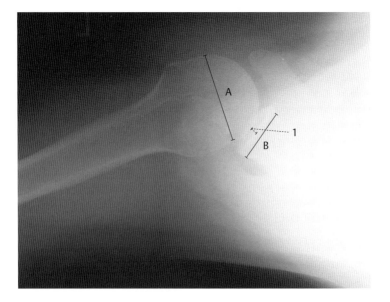

Checklist

Shape	• Spherical humeral head
	• Normal shape and size of glenoid (see below)
	• Coracoid process (clear projection)
	• Acromioclavicular joint
Position	• Articulation in the joint
	• Normal width of joint space (see below)
	• Coverage by the acromion
Structure	• Mineralization
	• Normal trabeculation
	• Sharp delineation of trabecular pattern
	• No circumscribed densities or lucencies
	• Epiphyseal plates (open/closed)
Joint	• Contours: cortex smooth and sharp
	• No contour defects or discontinuities
	• No marginal osteophytes or sclerotic areas
	• Normal distance from acromion
	• Intra-articular or periarticular calcifications?
Other bones	• Contours: cortex smooth and sharp (especially the humeral shaft)
	• Normal cortical bone thickness
	• No contour defects or discontinuities
Soft tissues	• No swelling
	• No foreign bodies
	• Fat pad apposed to the bone
	• No calcifications (vascular, intra-articular or periarticular, at tendon attachments)

Important Data

1. Width of joint space = 4–6 mm
2. Glenohumeral index: B/A × 100
   50 = normal

Tangential Shoulder View (Biceps Tendon Canal)

The humeral head and tuberosities display a normal shape. Mineralization, bone structure, and cortical margins are unremarkable.

The bicipital groove is sharply defined and shows a normal depth and configuration. The groove is clearly projected with no sign of abnormalities.

Other imaged skeletal structures are unremarkable.

There are no soft-tissue abnormalities.

Interpretation

The bicipital groove appears normal.

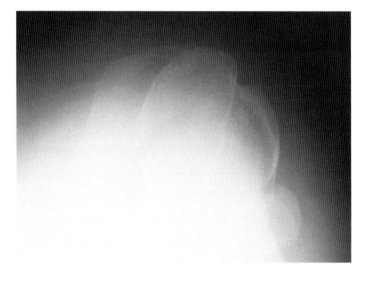

Checklist

Humeral head

Shape	• Spherical humeral head
	• Clear delineation of greater and lesser tuberosities
Structure	• Mineralization
	• Cancellous trabeculae are sharply defined and show a normal arrangement
	• No circumscribed densities or lucencies
	• Epiphyseal plates (open/closed)
Contours	• Cortex smooth and sharp
	• No contour defects or discontinuities
	• No marginal osteophytes or sclerotic areas

Bicipital groove

Shape	• U-shaped
	• Depth
Contours	• Cortex smooth and sharp
	• No contour defects or discontinuities
	• No osteophytes on the tuberosities
	• No narrowing of the groove
	• No calcifications in the groove
Other bones	• Acromion, clavicle
	• Shape, structure, contours
	• No contour defects or masses
Soft tissues	• No swelling or masses
	• No foreign bodies
	• No calcifications

Humerus, Biplane Views

The imaged skeletal structures show an anatomically normal shape and position with proper mineralization and bone structure. The cortex has smooth, sharp contours and is not thinned or thickened.

The articular surfaces are normally shaped and congruent and have smooth, sharp borders. The joint space is of normal width. There are no intra-articular or periarticular calcifications.

The soft-tissue envelope is unremarkable.

Interpretation

The humerus and imaged portions of the elbow joint appear normal.

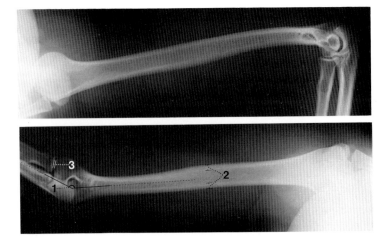

Checklist

Shape	• Long tubular bone
	• No angulation
	• Size
Position	• Elbow carrying angle (see below)
Structure	• Mineralization
	• Normal trabeculation
	• Sharp delineation of the trabecular pattern
	• No circumscribed lucencies or densities
	• Harmonious width of medullary cavities
	• Epiphyseal plates (open/closed)
Contours	• Cortex smooth and sharp
	• Normal cortical bone thickness (see below)
	• No contour defects or discontinuities
	• No periosteal reaction or elevation
Joint	• Shape (congruent)
	• Articular surfaces (smooth with sharp margins)
	• Width of joint space (see below)
	• No intra-articular or periarticular calcifications
Soft tissues	• Intact
	• No swelling
	• No foreign bodies
	• Fat pad apposed to the bone (especially near the joint)
	• No calcifications (vascular or at tendon attachments)

Important Data

1. Elbow carrying angle = 162°
2. Total cortical bone thickness (at mid-humerus) = 5–10 mm
3. Width of elbow joint space = 3 mm

Humerus, Transthoracic View

The imaged portions of the humerus have a normal shape, with normal articulation of the humeral head. There are no gross abnormalities of bone structure. Both the head and shaft of the humerus show intact cortical margins.

Other evaluable bones comprising the shoulder joint are unremarkable.

Interpretation

The humerus and humeral head appear normal, with no evidence of a fracture or other abnormalities.

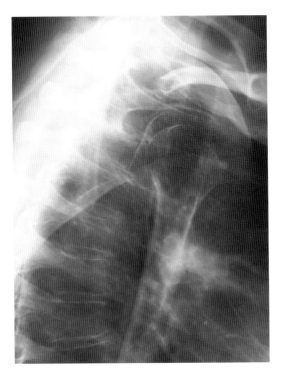

Checklist

Shape	● Spherical humeral head
	● Humeral shaft (straight)
Position	● Normal articulation
	● Coverage by the acromion
Structure	● No gross abnormalities (increased density or lysis; fine structure cannot be evaluated!)
Joint	● Contours: cortex smooth and sharp
	● No contour defects or discontinuities
	● No marginal osteophytes or sclerotic areas
	● Normal distance from the acromion
	● Intra-articular or periarticular calcifications?
Rest of skeleton	● Contours: cortex smooth and sharp (especially along the humeral shaft)
	● Normal cortical bone thickness
	● No contour defects or discontinuities
Soft tissues	● No gross abnormalities

Elbow Joint, Biplane Views

The distal humerus, radius, and ulna show a normal shape and position, also proper mineralization and bone structure. The cortical bone displays normal thickness and contours.

The articular surfaces have a normal configuration, smooth, sharp borders, and joint spaces of normal width. There are no intra-articular or periarticular calcifications.

The soft-tissue envelope is unremarkable.

Interpretation

The elbow appears normal.

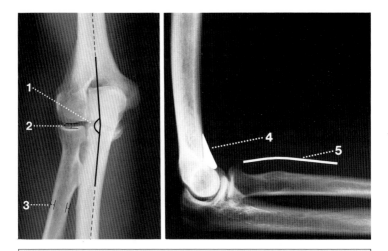

Important Data

1. Elbow carrying angle = 162°
2. Width of elbow joint space: ca. 3 cm
3. Total cortical bone thickness (in proximal radius) = 5–8 mm
4. Distal humeral fat pad (DHF):
   (**a**) Anterior DHF: proximal to coronoid fossa, ca. 5 mm thick, adjoins the bone
   (**b**) Posterior DHF: normally not visualized
5. Supinator fat plane: parallel to proximal radius, ca. 3–4 cm long and 2–3 mm thick

Checklist

Shape	• Humerus
	• Ulna
	• Radius (especially the radial head), olecranon
Position	• Carrying angle
	• Articulation of radial head, coronoid process, and olecranon
Structure	• Mineralization
	• Normal trabeculation
	• Sharp delineation of the trabecular pattern
	• No circumscribed lucencies or densities
	• Normal width of medullary cavities
	• Epiphyseal plates (open/closed)
Contours (bone)	• Cortex smooth and sharp
	• Normal cortical bone thickness (see below)
	• No contour defects or discontinuities
	• No periosteal reaction or elevation
	• No subperiosteal lucencies
	• No spurring
Joint	• Shape (congruent)
	• Cortex smooth and sharp
	• Normal cortical bone thickness (no circumscribed thickening or thinning)
	• No contour defects or discontinuities
	• Articular surfaces (smooth, sharp, congruent)
	• No impressions or sclerosis
	• No marginal osteophytes
	• Joint space (congruent, width—see below)
	• No intra-articular or periarticular calcifications
Soft tissues	• Intact
	• No swelling
	• No foreign bodies
	• Fat pad apposed to the bone (especially near the joint)
	• No calcifications (vascular or at tendon attachments)

Axial Elbow View

The capitulum and trochlea of the humerus and the olecranon have an anatomically normal shape and position, with proper mineralization and bone structure. The cortical margins are smooth and sharp with no abnormal contour defects.

The cubital tunnel presents a normal shape and depth.

There is no evidence of calcifications or radiopaque foreign bodies, and the soft tissues are unremarkable.

Interpretation

The cubital tunnel appears normal.

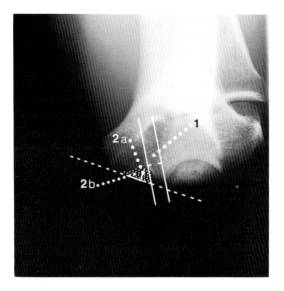

Checklist

Shape	•	Trochlea
	•	Normal shape of ulnar groove (no posttraumatic changes)
	•	Normal depth of cubital tunnel (see below)
Position	•	Position of olecranon in the trochlea, position of radius
Structure	•	Mineralization
	•	Sharp delineation of cancellous trabecular structure
	•	No circumscribed lucencies or densities
Contours	•	Cortex smooth and sharp (especially on articular surfaces)
	•	Normal cortical bone thickness
	•	No contour defects (especially in the lateral and medial epicondyles and olecranon)
	•	No marginal osteophytes (especially at the medial trochlear border)
	•	Normal width of distal elbow joint space
Soft tissues	•	Intact
	•	No swelling
	•	No intra-articular bony foreign bodies, no ossicles in the cubital tunnel
	•	No calcifications

Important Data

1. *Medial incongruity:* distance between a line tangent to the medial side of the trochlea and a parallel line at the media border of the olecranon should be less than 5 mm
2. *Cubital tunnel*
   (**a**) Depth: ca. 6.8 (3.6–11.1) mm
   (**b**) Area: ca. 0.88 cm^2

Forearm, Biplane Views

Both projections of the forearm show normal shape and position of the imaged bones, with normal mineralization and bone structure. The cortical margins are smooth and sharp with no pathological contour defects. Cortical bone thickness is normal.

The proximal and distal articular surfaces have an anatomically normal shape. The articulating surfaces are smooth and congruent, and all joint spaces are of normal width. There is no sign of intra-articular or peri-articular calcifications.

The soft tissues are unremarkable.

Interpretation

The forearm appears normal.

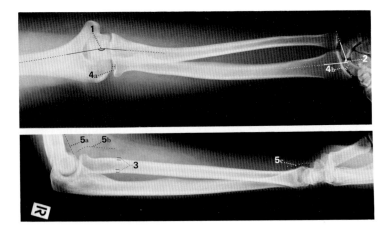

Checklist

Shape	• Radius, ulna: shape, size
Position	• Parallel
	• Radioulnar distance
	• Normal angles (see below)
Structure	• Mineralization
	• Normal trabeculation
	• Sharp delineation of trabecular pattern
	• No circumscribed lucencies or densities
	• Harmonious width of medullary cavities
	• Epiphyseal plates (open/closed)
Contours	• Cortex smooth and sharp
	• Normal cortical bone thickness (see below)
	• No contour defects or discontinuities
	• No periosteal reaction or elevation
	• No spurring
Joint	• Shape of articular surfaces (congruent)
	• Contours (smooth and sharp)
	• No marginal osteophytes
	• Width of joint space (see below)
	• No intra-articular or periarticular calcifications
	• Accessory bones at typical location
Soft tissues	• Intact, no swelling
	• No foreign bodies
	• Fat pad apposed to the bone (see below)
	• No calcifications (vascular or at tendon attachments)

Important Data

1. *Elbow carrying angle* = 162°
2. *Angle of wrist joint line* in AP projection = 72–95°
3. *Total cortical bone thickness* (in proximal radius) = 5–8 mm
4. *Width of joint spaces:*
   (**a**) Elbow joint = 3 mm
   (**b**) Radiocarpal joint = 2–2.5 mm
5. *Fat pads:*
   (**a**) Distal humeral fat pad
   (**b**) Supinator fat plane
   (**c**) Presence of pronator quadratus sign (compared with opposite side)

Hand, Biplane Views

The phalanges, metacarpals, and carpal bones are normal in shape, size, number, and position. They exhibit proper mineralization and bone structure. The cortical margins are smooth and sharp with no abnormal contour defects. Cortical bone thickness is normal. The articular surfaces have an anatomically normal shape and smooth borders. The joint spaces are of normal width. There is no sign of intra-articular or periarticular calcifications.

The soft tissues are unremarkable.

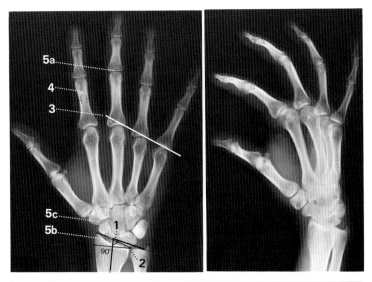

Important Data

1. *Angle of wrist joint line* in AP projection = 72–95°
2. *Angle of radiocarpal joint line* in AP projection = 30°
3. *Metacarpal sign:* a line tangent to the distal ends of the 4th and 5th metacarpals does not touch the 3d metacarpal
4. *Total cortical bone thickness* (in proximal phalanx of index finger): 4–5 mm
5. *Width of joint spaces:*
   (**a**) Interphalangeal joints = 1–2 mm
   (**b**) Radiocarpal joint = 2–2.5 mm
   (**c**) Intercarpal joint = 1.5–2 mm

Interpretation

The bones of the hand appear normal.

Checklist

Shape	• Shape of hand bones
	• Number (5 rays; 5 metacarpals; 5 proximal, middle, and distal phalanges; 8 carpal bones)
Position	• Normal angle of wrist joint line relative to radial axis (see below)
	• No metacarpal sign (due to growth disturbance, see below)
	• Normal distance between the metacarpal heads (2/3 > 4/5 ≥ 3/4)
	• Normal radiocarpal joint angle (see below)
Structure	• Mineralization
	• Normal trabeculation
	• Sharp delineation of trabecular pattern
	• No circumscribed lucencies or densities
	• Normal width of medullary canals
	• Epiphyseal plates (open/closed)
Contours	• Cortex smooth and sharp
	• Normal cortical bone thickness (see below)
	• No contour defects or discontinuities
	• No periosteal reaction or elevation
	• No sclerosis
Joints	• Articular surfaces (interphalangeal, metacarpophalangeal and carpometacarpal joint spaces): shape, contours (smooth and sharp)
	• Normal width of joint spaces (see below)
	• No marginal osteophytes
	• No sclerosis or erosions (including subchondral zone)
	• No intra-articular or periarticular calcifications
	• Accessory bones at typical location
Soft tissues	• Intact
	• Normal thickness
	• No foreign bodies
	• Fat planes apposed to the bone (especially near joints)
	• No calcifications (vascular or at tendon attachments)

Wrist, Biplane Views

The bones of the wrist appear normal in shape, size, and number. They show a normal relationship to one another, to the metacarpals, and to the radius and ulna.

Mineralization and bone structure are normal.

The cortical margins are smooth and sharp with no pathological contour defects.

The articular surfaces are normally shaped and have joint spaces of normal width. Imaged portions of the radius, ulna, and metacarpals are unremarkable.

The soft tissues are intact and contain no radiopaque foreign bodies or calcifications.

Interpretation

The wrist appears normal.

Checklist

Shape	• Number (8 carpal bones)
	• Size of carpal bones
	• Shape of radius, ulna, carpal bones, and metacarpals
Position	• Normal angle of wrist joint line relative to radial axis (see below)
	• Normal radiocarpal joint angle (see below)
Structure	• Mineralization
	• Normal trabeculation
	• Sharp delineation of trabecular pattern
	• No circumscribed lucencies or densities (e.g., patchy, cystic, bandlike, diffuse)
	• Width of medullary canals
Contours	• Cortex smooth and sharp
	• No contour defects or discontinuities
	• No periosteal reactions
	• No sclerosis or erosions
Joints	• Intercarpal joints:
	— Shape
	— Smooth, sharp margins
	— No discontinuities
	— Normal width of joint space (see below)
	• Radiocarpal joint:
	— Shape (plateaulike boundary)
	— Smooth, sharp margins
	— Normal width of joint space (see below)
	— Normal position of radius and ulna
	— Normal radial and ulnar styloids
	• Carpometacarpal joints:
	— Shape
	— Smooth, sharp margins
	— No discontinuities
	— No intra-articular or periarticular foreign bodies
	— Normal width of joint space (see below)
	— No marginal osteophytes
	— No subchondral sclerosis or erosion
	• *Accessory bones* at typical location
Other bones	• Radius, ulna, metacarpals (position, structure, contours)
Soft tissues	• Normal thickness, no foreign bodies
	• Fat planes apposed to the bone (especially near joints)
	• No calcifications (vascular or at tendon attachments)

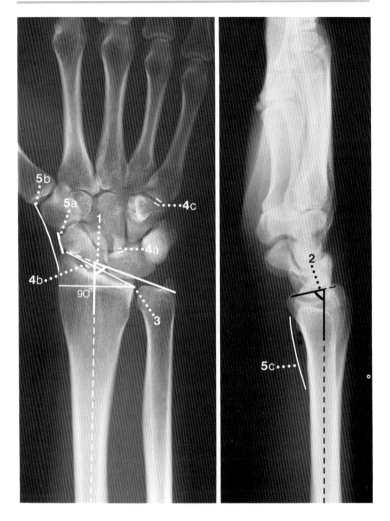

Important Data

1. *Angle of wrist joint line* in AP projection = 72–95°
2. *Angle of wrist joint line* in lateral projection = 79–94°
3. *Angle of radiocarpal joint line* in AP projection = ca. 30°
4. *Width of joint spaces:*
   (**a**) Intercarpal joint = 1.5–2 mm
   (**b**) Radiocarpal joint = 2–2.5 mm
   (**c**) Carpometacarpal joints = 1–2 mm
5. (**a**) Scaphoid fat stripe: just radial to scaphoid bone
   (**b**) Fat stripe of thumb-muscle tendon sheath
   (**c**) Pronator quadratus sign: distal palmar forearm

Carpal Tunnel View

The carpal and metacarpal bones that bound the carpal tunnel are normal in shape, size, number, and position. They show proper mineralization and bone structure.

The cortical margins are smooth and sharp with no pathological contour defects. The carpal tunnel does not contain visible accessory bones. The soft tissues appear normal and symmetrical. There are no radiopaque foreign bodies or calcifications.

Interpretation

The soft tissues of the carpal tunnel and its bony boundaries appear normal.

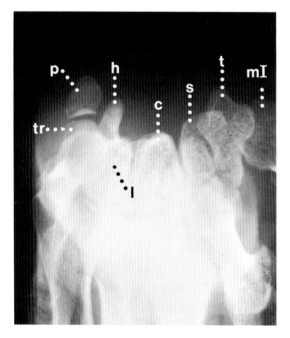

Checklist

Shape	• Carpal bones (number) from radial to ulnar side: trapezium, scaphoid, capitate, lunate, hamate (with hamulus), pisiform, and first metacarpal
	• No accessory bones in the carpal tunnel!
Position	• Compare with opposite side
	• No dislocation of carpal bones (especially the lunate)
Structure	• Mineralization
	• Sharp delineation of cancellous trabecular pattern
	• No circumscribed lucencies or densities
Contours	• Cortex smooth and sharp
	• No abnormal contour defects or discontinuities
	• No circumscribed density, excrescence, or sclerosis
	• Erosion (especially due to osteoarthritis or inflammation)
Soft tissues	• Intact skin (tangentially imaged)
	• No soft-tissue thickening or swelling (right–left discrepancy?)
	• No calcium deposits
	• No radiopaque foreign bodies

Important Data

Triquetral bone (tr)
Pisiform bone (p)
Hamulus of hamate bone (h)
Lunate bone (l)
Capitate bone (c)
Scaphoid bone (s)
Trapezium bone (t)
First metacarpal bone (ml)

Scaphoid View

The scaphoid bone is normal in shape, size, and position. It displays proper mineralization and bone structure. The cortical margins are smooth and sharp with no abnormal contour defects.

The articular surfaces are normally shaped and have smooth, sharp borders. Other imaged bones are unremarkable. There are no foreign bodies or calcifications.

Interpretation

The scaphoid bone appears normal.

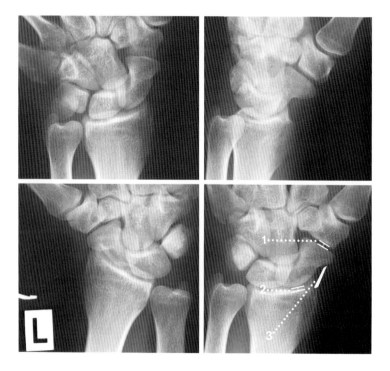

Checklist

Shape	• Size (scaphoid is largest bone in proximal row)
	• Shape
	• Consists of one part
Position	• Articulates with the radius, lunate, trapezium, trapezoid, and capitate
Structure	• Mineralization
	• Normal trabeculation
	• Sharp delineation of trabecular pattern
	• No circumscribed lucencies or densities (patchy, cystic, diffuse, bandlike) (most fractures occur in the central [~ 50%] or proximal [~ 37%] part of the bone)
Contours	• Cortex smooth and sharp
	• No abnormal contour defects or discontinuities
	• No bony excrescences
	• No flake fracture (especially on the radial aspect)
	• No sclerosis
Joint	• Shape of articular surfaces
	• Contours (smooth, sharp borders)
	• Normal width of joint spaces (see below)
	• No marginal osteophytes
	• No intra-articular or periarticular foreign bodies
	• Accessory bones at typical location
	• Fat stripe not displaced (see below)
Soft tissues	• No foreign bodies or calcifications

Important Data

Width of joint spaces:
1. Intercarpal joints = 1.5–2 mm
2. Radiocarpal joint = 2–2.5 mm
3. Scaphoid fat stripe: just radial to the scaphoid bone

Special View of the Pisiform Bone

The shape, size, and position of the pisiform bone are normal. It shows proper mineralization and bone structure. The cortical margins are smooth and sharp with no abnormal contour defects.

The articular surfaces are normally shaped and have smooth, sharp borders.

Other imaged bones are unremarkable, especially the lunate, scaphoid, hamate, and trapezium. There is no evidence of accessory bones.

There are no foreign bodies or calcifications.

Interpretation

The pisiform bone appears normal.

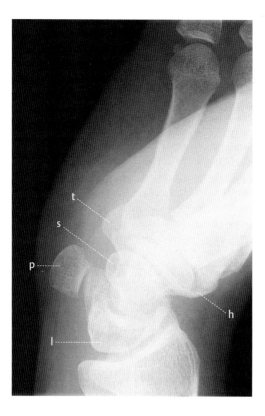

Checklist

Shape	• Size
	• Shape
	• Consists of one part
Position	• Articulates with the triquetral and hamate bones
	• Pisiform is not displaced by capitate excrescences
Structure	• Mineralization
	• Normal trabeculation
	• Sharp delineation of trabecular pattern
	• No circumscribed lucencies or densities (patchy, cystic, diffuse, bandlike)
Contours	• Cortex smooth and sharp
	• No abnormal contour defects or discontinuities
	• No bony excrescences
	• No flake fracture
	• No sclerosis
Joint	• Shape of articular surfaces
	• Contours (smooth, sharp borders)
	• Normal width of joint spaces
	• No marginal osteophytes
	• No intra-articular or periarticular foreign bodies
	• No accessory elements distal to pisiform bone (external lunate bone) between the pisiform and triquetral
Soft tissues	• No foreign bodies
	• No calcifications
	• No calcium deposits on the volar aspect (e.g., flexor carpi ulnaris tendinitis or calcifying periarthritis)

Important Data

The following carpal bones are visible in the pisiform view:
Pisiform (p)
Lunate (l)
Scaphoid (s)
Hamate (h)
Trapezium (t)

Individual Fingers, Biplane Views

The phalanges are of normal shape (including the distal phalanx, within the range of variation) and show proper axial alignment.

Mineralization and bone structure appear normal. The cortical margins are smooth and sharp with no pathological contour defects. Cortical thickness is normal. The lanula is intact.

The articular surfaces are normally shaped, have smooth margins, and are congruent. The joint spaces are of normal width throughout. There are no intra-articular or periarticular calcifications.

The soft-tissue envelope is unremarkable.

Interpretation

The finger appears normal.

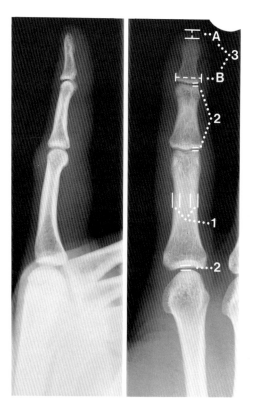

Checklist

Shape	• Shape
	• Size
	• Number of members (metacarpal + proximal, middle, and distal phalanges)
Position	• Straight axis (no lateral deviation)
Structure	• Mineralization
	• Normal trabeculation
	• Sharp delineation of trabecular pattern
	• No circumscribed lucencies or densities
	• Harmonious width of medullary canals
	• Epiphyseal plates (open/closed)
Contours	• Cortex smooth and sharp
	• Normal cortical bone thickness (see below)
	• No contour defects or discontinuities
	• No periosteal reaction or elevation
	• No sclerosis
	• No dissection of cortical bone
	• Lanula intact
Joints	• Shape of articular surfaces (congruent)
	• Contours (smooth, sharp)
	• No erosions or cysts
	• No osteophytes
	• Width of joint spaces (see below)
	• No intra-articular or periarticular calcifications
	• No isolated bone fragments
	• Accessory bones at typical location
Soft tissues	• Intact
	• Normal thickness (see below)
	• No foreign bodies
	• No calcifications (vascular or at tendon attachments)

Important Data

1. *Total cortical bone thickness* (in proximal phalanx of index finger) = 4–5 mm
2. *Width of joint spaces* = 1–2 mm
3. *Yune soft-tissue index:* thickness of fingertip (A)/width of lanula (B) = at least 25%

The Lower Extremity

Full-Length Standing Radiograph

The leg displays a normal shape and position, particularly with respect to its anatomical and mechanical axes. Normal articulation is observed in the hip, knee, and ankle joints. The long tubular bones are normally shaped and show proper mineralization and bone structure. The cortical margins are smooth and sharp with no pathological contour defects or discontinuities.

The hip joint is unremarkable. The femoral head is well rounded and is adequately covered by the acetabular roof.

The articular surfaces of the knee joint are congruent.

The ankle joint is morphologically normal, with a normal appearance of the ankle mortise.

All the joint spaces display a normal width. There is no sign of intra-articular or periarticular calcifications.

The soft-tissue envelope is unremarkable.

Interpretation

The lower extremity appears normal.

Checklist

Position	• Femoral head, femur, knee joint, ankle joint: mechanical and anatomical axes (see below)
Long tubular bones	• Shape (normal proportions of femur, tibia, and fibula; no angular deformity)
	• Structure (mineralization, cancellous trabeculae)
	• Contours (cortex smooth, no abnormal contour defects or discontinuities)
	• Normal cortical bone thickness
	• Epiphyseal plates (open/closed)
Hip	• Acetabular roof (coverage)
	• Femoral head (roundness)
	• Shape (joint congruity)
	• Width of joint space
Knee	• Shape (congruity of articular surfaces)
	• Structure
	• Contours (cortex smooth and intact, no marginal osteophytes or sclerosis)
	• Width of joint space (symmetry)
	• Patella (position, shape)
Ankle joint	• Shape (development of ankle mortise, congruity of articular surfaces)
	• Contours (cortex smooth and intact, no significant marginal osteophytes or sclerosis)
	• Width of joint space
Soft tissues	• Intact
	• No swelling
	• No foreign bodies
	• No calcifications (intra-articular or periarticular, vascular, at tendon attachments)

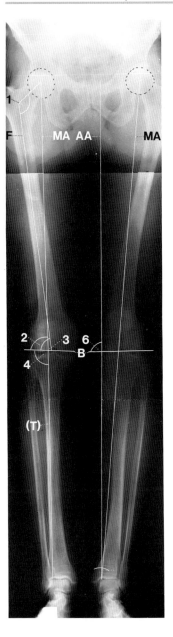

Important Data

1. *CCD angle:* 120°–130°
   Mechanical axis (MA): from the center of the femoral head to the center of the ankle joint.
   Normally, MA runs through the center of the knee joint (if angular deformity exists, the angle between MA and a line from the center of the femoral head to the center of the knee joint should be determined).
2. Mechanical axis (MA)/knee baseline (B) = ca. 87°
3. Femoral shaft axis (F)/knee baseline (B) = ca. 81°
4. Knee baseline (B)/tibial shaft axis (T) = ca. 93° (tibial shaft axis [T] is from center of knee to center of ankle joint)
5. Mechanical axis (MA)/anatomic axis (AA) = 5–7°
6. Anatomic axis (AA)/knee baseline (B) = 90°

Hip, Biplane Views

The hip joint has an anatomically normal shape with proper articulation of the femoral head in the acetabulum. The CCD angle is within normal limits.

Mineralization and bone structure appear normal. The cortical margins are smooth and sharp with no pathological contour defects.

The articular surfaces are smooth and normally configured, and the joint space is of normal width throughout. The articulating surfaces are congruent, and the femoral head is well covered by the roof of the acetabulum.

The soft tissues are unremarkable.

Interpretation

The hip joint appears normal.

Checklist

Shape
- Acetabular roof
- Normal round shape of femoral head
- Normal appearance of greater and lesser trochanters

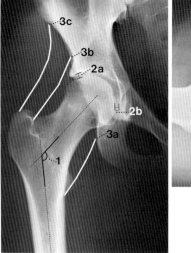
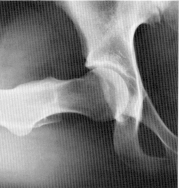

Position	• Femoral head centered in acetabulum
	• Normal CCD angle (see below)
Structure	• Mineralization
	• Normal trabeculation
	• Sharp delineation of trabecular pattern
	• No circumscribed lucencies or densities
	• Normal trajectorial pattern from head to shaft
	• Normal width of medullary canals
	• Epiphyseal plates (open/closed)
Contours	• Cortex smooth and sharp, normal cortical thickness
	• No contour defects or discontinuities
	• No periosteal reaction or elevation
Joint	• Morphology
	• Smooth fovea
	• Femoral head coverage
	• Articular surfaces (smooth, sharp, congruent)
	• No sclerosis, subcortical lucencies, or subchondral densities
	• Width of joint space (see below)
	• No marginal osteophytes (fovea, femoral head, acetabular roof)
	• No intraarticular or periarticular calcifications
Soft tissues	• Intact
	• No swelling
	• No foreign bodies
	• Fat pad apposed to the bone (especially near the joint, see below)
	• No calcifications (vascular or at tendon attachments)

Important Data

1. *CCD angle:* 120–130°
2. *Width of joint space*:
   (**a**) Superior portion: 3–4 mm
   (**b**) Medial portion: 4–5 mm
3. *Fat stripes:*
   (**a**) Medial to iliopsoas muscle
   (**b**) Medial to gluteus minimus
   (**c**) Between the gluteal muscles (inconstant)

Contour Views of the Femoral Head

The anterior and posterior surfaces of the femoral head present a normal shape. The cortical borders of the femoral head are smooth, sharply defined, and of normal thickness with no pathologic contour defects. There are no abnormal lucencies or densities and no marginal osteophytes.

The joint space is of normal width. The articular surfaces of the femur and acetabulum are congruent, with good coverage of the femoral head. The contours of the acetabulum are smooth.

Visible portions of the femur, ischium, pubis, and iliac wing are unremarkable.

The soft tissues appear normal.

Interpretation

The hip joint appears normal. In particular, the anterior and posterior surfaces of the femoral head show no abnormalities.

Checklist

Shape
- The anterior surface (Schneider I) and posterior surface (Schneider II) of the femoral head are clearly projected

Schneider I projection of the femoral head

Schneider II projection of the femoral head

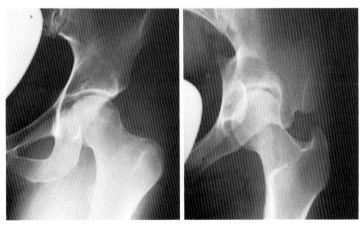

- Shape: round (Schneider I), elliptical (Schneider II)
- Contours: smooth and sharp, normal cortical thickness
- No contour defects or discontinuities
- No impressions
- Smooth outlines of the fovea
- No marginal osteophytes
- No abnormal sclerosis
- No circumscribed (subcortical) lucencies or (subchondral) densities
- Normal bone structure

Hip joint
- Congruity of the articular surfaces
- Femoral head coverage
- Contours of the acetabulum (smooth, sharply defined)
- No increased sclerosis or lucencies
- No marginal osteophytes (fovea, femoral head, acetabular roof)
- No intra-articular or periarticular calcifications

Femur
- *Femoral neck:*
  - Smooth contours with no defects or discontinuities
  - Normal trajectorial pattern
  - Structure (mineralization, trabeculation)
  - No abnormal lucencies or densities
- *Greater trochanter* (best seen in the Schneider II projection):
  - Shape
  - Contours (no defects)
  - Structure (mineralization, trabeculation)
  - Calcifications at tendon attachments

Other bones
- Ischium (best seen in the Schneider II projection)
- Pubis (if visualized)
- Portions of iliac wing (if visualized)
- Shape
- Structure (mineralization, trabeculation)
- Contours (no defects or discontinuities)

Soft tissues
- Intact
- No swelling
- No foreign bodies
- Fat pad apposed to the bone (especially near the joint)
- No calcifications (vascular or at tendon attachments)

Femur, Biplane Views

The imaged skeletal structures display an anatomically normal shape and position.

Mineralization and bone structure appear normal. The cortical borders are smooth and sharp with no defects or discontinuities. The articular surfaces of the knee joint are normally shaped, smoothly marginated, and congruent. The joint space is of normal width throughout. There are no intra-articular or periarticular calcifications.

The soft-tissue envelope is unremarkable.

Interpretation

The femur appears normal.

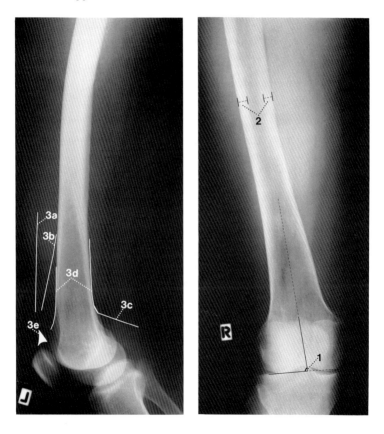

Checklist

Shape	• Long tubular bone
Position	• Normal angle between the femur and knee joint (see below)
Structure	• Mineralization
	• Normal trabeculation
	• Sharp delineation of the trabecular pattern
	• No contour defects or discontinuities
	• Normal width of medullary cavities
	• Epiphyseal plates (open/closed)
Contours	• Cortex smooth and sharp
	• Normal cortical bone thickness (see below)
	• No contour defects or discontinuities
	• No periosteal reaction or elevation (especially over the medial condyle)
Joint	• Shape of articular surfaces (congruent)
	• Contours (smooth, sharp)
	• Joint space (see below)
	• No intra-articular or periarticular calcifications
	• No isolated bone fragments
Soft tissues	• Intact, no swelling
	• Fat pad apposed to the bone (especially near the joint, see below)
	• No calcifications (vascular or at tendon attachments)
	• No foreign bodies

Important Data

1. *Angle between femoral shaft and knee joint line*: 81° (75–85°)
2. *Total cortical bone thickness* = ca. 20 mm
3. *Fat planes:*
   Muscular fat planes:
   (**a**) Rectus femoris,
   (**b**) Vastus intermedius,
   (**c**) Border of gastrocnemius
   (**d**) Fat planes along the femoral metaphysis (anterior and posterior fat planes are normally apposed to the bone)
   (**e**) Suprapatellar fat pad

Knee Joint, Biplane Views

The knee joint displays a normal position and morphology, with proper bone structure and mineralization. The articular surfaces are smooth and congruent, and the width of the joint space is normal. The cortical boundaries of the femur and tibia are smooth and sharp.

The patella has a normal shape and shows proper articulation with the femur. Its articular surfaces present smooth margins. There are no intra-articular or periarticular calcifications or foreign bodies.

The soft tissues are unremarkable.

Interpretation

The knee joint appears normal.

Checklist

Shape	• Femoral condyles
	• Tibial plateau
Position	• Physiological valgus (see below)
	• Tibia centered below the joint
Structure	• Mineralization
	• Normal trabeculation
	• Sharp delineation of the trabecular pattern

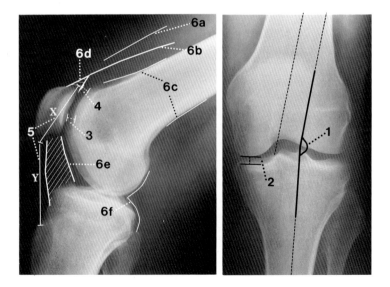

	•	No circumscribed lucencies or densities (especially in the medial epicondyle)
Joint	•	Shape (congruity)
	•	Contours: cortex smooth and sharp, normal cortical thickness
	•	No contour defects, impressions, or discontinuities
	•	No sclerosis or marginal osteophytes
	•	Two intercondylar tubercles (intact contours, no peaking)
	•	Width of joint space (see below)
Femur, tibia	•	Cortex smooth and sharp
(contours)	•	Normal cortical thickness
	•	No contour defects or discontinuities (notching of the lateral condyle is normal in the lateral view and helps distinguish it from the medial condyle)
	•	No bony excrescences (especially on the medial epi-condyle)
	•	Tibial tuberosity is contiguous to the tibia (sharply marginated, not fragmented)
	•	Epiphyseal plates (open/closed)
Patella	•	Shape, no dysplasia (see below)
	•	Articulation, articular surfaces (smooth, sharp)
	•	No sclerosis or marginal osteophytes
	•	Width of joint space (see below)
	•	No foreign bodies
Soft tissues	•	No swelling or foreign bodies
	•	Fat pad apposed to the bone (especially near the joint, see below)
	•	No calcifications (vascular or at tendon attachments)

Important Data

1. *Physiologic valgus of the knee:* 173°
2. *Width of knee joint space:* 3–5 mm
3. *Width of femoropatellar joint space:* < 5 mm
4. *Base of suprapatellar bursa:* < 5 mm
5. *Patellar dysplasia:* Y/X = 0.8–1.2
6. *Fat planes:*
   Muscular fat planes:
   (**a**) Rectus femoris
   (**b**) Vastus intermedius
   (**c**) Fat planes along the femoral metaphysis (anterior and posterior fat planes are normally apposed to the bone)
   (**d**) Suprapatellar fat pad
   (**e**) Infrapatellar fat pad
   (**f**) Popliteal fat plane

Knee Joint, Tunnel View

The knee joint shows normal position and morphology. Its articular surfaces are smooth and congruent, and they have sharp margins with no contour defects. The intercondylar tubercles and the intercondylar notch of the femur appear normal. The joint space is of normal width with no intra-articular loose bodies or calcifications.

The femur, tibia, and fibula are unremarkable.

The soft tissues are normal.

Interpretation

The knee joint space and cruciate ligament region appear normal.

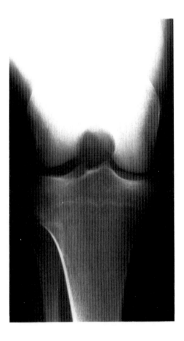

Checklist

Shape	• Femoral condyles
	• Intercondylar notch
	• Tibial plateau
	• Intercondylar tubercles
Position	• Articulation
	• Congruity of articular surfaces
Joint	• Cortex (smooth, sharp)
Contours	• Normal cortical thickness
	• No contour defects, impressions, or discontinuities
	• No depressions (e.g., from a joint mouse on the medial condyle)
	• Marginal osteophytes (e.g., osteoarthritis, Rauber sign)
	• No areas of subchondral decalcification or sclerosis
	• Intercondylar tubercles (intact contours, no peaking)
	• Intercondylar notch (smooth outline, no osteophytes or calcifications)
Joint space	• Width (uniform)
	• No intra-articular loose bodies
	• No intra-articular or periarticular calcifications (menisci, cruciate ligaments)
Other bones	• Mineralization
	• Trabecular structure (lucencies, densities)
Contours	• Cortex (smooth, intact, no abnormal sclerosis)
	• Normal cortical thickness
	• No bony excrescences (e.g., Stieda shadow)
	• Epiphyseal plates (open/closed)
Soft tissues	• Intact
	• No swelling
	• No foreign bodies
	• Fat pad apposed to the bone (especially near the joint)
	• No calcifications (vascular or at tendon attachments)

Patella, 30°, 60°, and 90° Views

These views demonstrate an anatomically normal shape of the patella and femoral condyles and a normal patellar position.

Bone structure and mineralization are normal. The cortical borders are smooth, sharp, and of normal thickness with no pathological contour defects.

The articulating surfaces of the patella and femur are smooth and sharply defined, and the femoropatellar joint space is of normal width. There are no intra-articular or periarticular calcifications.

The soft-tissue envelope is unremarkable.

Interpretation

The patella and femoropatellar joint appear normal.

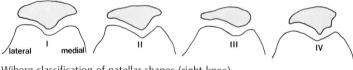

Wiberg classification of patellar shapes (right knee)

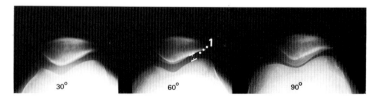

Checklist

Shape	•	Wiberg type I–IV
	•	Femoral condyles (lateral condyle is usually larger)
Position	•	Articulation of the patella in the femoral trochlea
Structure	•	Mineralization
	•	Normal trabeculation
	•	Sharp delineation of trabecular pattern
	•	No circumscribed lucencies or densities (especially in the medial patellar facet and femoral condyle)
Contours	•	Cortex smooth and sharp (in all views!)
	•	No contour defects or discontinuities
	•	No sclerosis
	•	No marginal osteophytes
	•	No bony excrescences (course of tendons)
Joint	•	Shape of articular surfaces (congruity)
	•	Patella and femur: smooth, sharp surface outlines (in all views!)
	•	Width of joint space (see below)
	•	No intra-articular or periarticular calcifications
Femur	•	Condyles (shape, structure, contours)
Soft tissues	•	Intact coverage
	•	No swelling
	•	No foreign bodies
	•	No calcifications (vascular or at tendon attachments)

Important Data

1. *Width of femoropatellar joint space:* < 5 mm

Tibia, Biplane Views

The bones displayed in these projections are properly shaped and positioned. The ankle mortise shows a normal configuration.

Mineralization and bone structure are unremarkable. The cortical margins are smooth and sharp with no abnormal contour defects. Cortical bone thickness is normal. The articular surfaces show an anatomically normal shape and smooth margins. The joint spaces are of normal width. There are no intra-articular or periarticular calcifications.

The soft-tissue envelope is unremarkable.

Interpretation

The tibia appears normal.

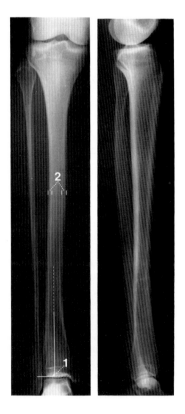

Checklist

Shape	● Two long tubular bones (tibia and fibula)
	● Configuration of the ankle mortise
Position	● Distance between the tibia and fibula
	● Angle between the tibial axis and joint line (Johnson angle) (see below)
Structure	● Mineralization
	● Normal trabeculation
	● Sharp delineation of the trabecular pattern
	● No circumscribed lucencies or densities
	● Normal width of the medullary cavities
	● Epiphyseal plates (open/closed)
Contours	● Cortex smooth and sharp
	● Normal cortical thickness (see below)
	● No contour defects or discontinuities
	● No periosteal reaction or elevation
	● No sclerosis
Joint	● Shape (congruity)
	● Contours of articular surfaces (smooth, sharp)
	● Joint space
	● Accessory bones at typical location
	● No isolated bone fragments
	● No intra-articular or periarticular calcifications
Soft tissues	● Intact
	● No swelling
	● Fat pad apposed to the bone (especially near the joint)
	● No calcifications (vascular, tendon attachments, interosseous membrane)
	● No radiopaque foreign bodies

Important Data

1. *Johnson angle* (between the tibial axis and ankle joint line) = ca. 90° (usually there is slight varus angulation)
2. *Total cortical bone thickness* (at mid-tibia) = 9–14 mm

Ankle Joint, Biplane Views

The bones about the ankle show a normal shape and position with a normal configuration of the ankle mortise.

The articular surfaces are congruent and have smooth, sharp surfaces. The joint space is of normal width.

Other imaged bones show normal mineralization and bone structure. They have smooth, sharp cortical borders with no abnormal contour defects. There are no intra-articular or periarticular calcifications.

The soft tissues are unremarkable.

Interpretation

The ankle joint appears normal.

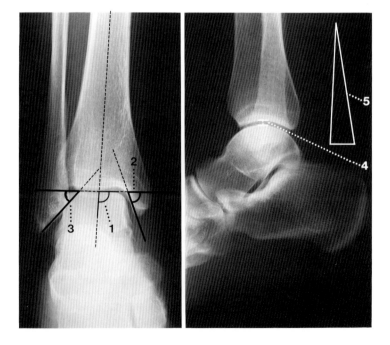

Checklist

Shape	● Configuration of the ankle mortise
	● Dorsal surface of the talus (rectangular)
Position	● Angle between the tibial axis and joint line (Johnson angle) (see below)
	● Tibial angle (see below)
	● Fibular angle (see below)
Joint	● Articular surfaces (smooth, sharp, congruent)
	● No contour defects or discontinuities
	● No sclerosis, lucency, or periosteal elevation
	● No marginal osteophytes
	● Width of joint space (see below)
	● Accessory bones at typical location
Other bones:	● Mineralization
Structure	● Trabeculation
	● Sharp delineation of trabecular pattern
	● No circumscribed lucencies or densities
	● Normal width of medullary cavities
	● Epiphyseal plates (open/closed)
Contours	● Smooth, sharp cortex
	● Normal cortical bone thickness
	● No contour defects or discontinuities
	● No sclerosis or cortical thinning
	● No bony excrescences or periosteal elevation
Soft tissues	● No swelling
	● No foreign bodies (extra-articular or intra-articular)
	● No displacement of soft-tissue planes (especially near the joint)
	● No calcifications (vascular, tendon attachments, interosseous membrane)
	● Normal achilles tendon shadow (see below)

Important Data

1. *Johnson angle* (between tibial axis and ankle joint line) = ca. 92°
2. *Tibial angle* = 45–65°
3. *Fibular angle* = 43–63°
4. *Width of joint space:* ankle joint = 3–4 mm
5. *Achilles tendon shadow:* triangle about 10–20 mm high and 2–4 mm wide at the base

Anterior and posterior borders of joint capsule: rarely identifiable unless the intra-articular volume is increased

Foot, Biplane Views

The pedal skeleton is normal in the shape, size, number, and position of the phalanges, metatarsal and tarsal bones. The pedal arch is normally developed, and the joint angles are normal. The bones display proper structure and mineralization.

The cortex is smooth, sharply defined, and of normal thickness with no abnormal contour defects.

The articular surfaces are normally shaped, smooth and sharply marginated and are separated by joint spaces of normal width. There are no intra-articular or periarticular calcifications.

The soft tissues are unremarkable.

Interpretation

The bones of the foot appear normal.

Checklist

Shape	• Number (5 rays; 5 metatarsals; 5 proximal, middle, and distal phalanges; 3 cuneiform bones; the cuboid, navicular, calcaneus, and talus)
Position	• Normal pedal arch (see below)
	• Normal shape of the calcaneus (see below)
	• Interrelationships of the tarsal bones
	• Proximal phalanx of big toe (see below)
Structure	• Mineralization
	• Trabeculation
	• Sharp delineation of trabecular pattern
	• No circumscribed lucencies or densities
	• Harmonious width of medullary cavities
	• Epiphyseal plates (open/closed)
Contours	• Cortex smooth and sharp
	• Normal cortical bone thickness (see below)
	• No contour defects or discontinuities
	• No periosteal reaction or elevation
	• No sclerosis
Joint	• Articular surfaces, tarsometatarsal and metatarso-phalangeal joint spaces: shape (congruity)
	• Contours (smooth and sharp)
	• Normal width of joint spaces (see below)
	• No marginal osteophytes
	• No subchondral sclerosis or erosion
	• No intra-articular or periarticular calcifications
	• Accessory bones at typical location
Soft tissues	• Intact
	• Normal thickness
	• No foreign bodies
	• Fat planes apposed to the bone (especially near joints)
	• No calcifications (vascular or at tendon attachments)

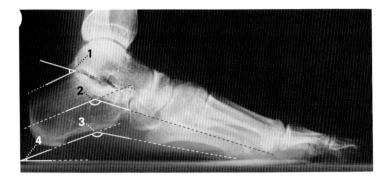

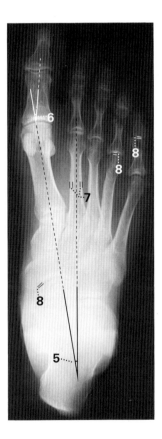

Important Data

1. *Angle between the calcaneal tuberosity and subtalar joint line =* 30–40°
2. *Angle between the calcaneal axis and the medial longitudinal axis of the foot =* 144 ± 5°

Pedal arch angles:

3. Angle between a tangent to the inferior border of the calcaneus and a tangent to the inferior border of the fifth metatarsal = 150–170°
4. Angle between a tangent to the inferior border of the calcaneus and the floor = 20–30°
5. Angle between the longitudinal axes of the first and second metatarsals = 7.4° ± 2.6° (>9° is suspicious for hallux valgus)
6. *Valgus angle of big toe:* <20° = normal
7. *Total cortical bone thickness* (midshaft, second metatarsal) = ca. 5 mm
8. *Width of joint spaces* = 2–2.5 mm (metatarsal and tarso-metatarsal joints) (interphalangeal joints: ca. 1–2 mm)

Calcaneus, Biplane Views

The calcaneus displays a normal shape and normal axes. It shows a normal relationship to the talus and cuboid, with no malalignment or deformity. Its mineralization and bone structure are normal, and there is sharp delineation of the cancellous trabeculae.

The cortex is smooth, sharply marginated, and of normal thickness with no abnormal contour defects.

The articular surfaces are congruent and are separated by joint spaces of normal width. Other imaged tarsal bones are unremarkable.

The soft tissues show no abnormalities.

Interpretation

The calcaneus appears normal.

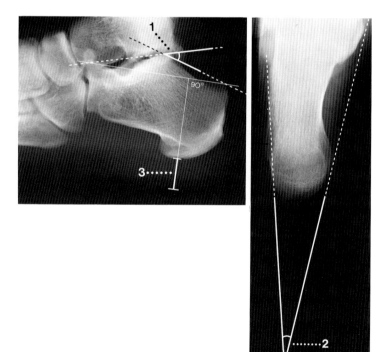

Checklist

Shape	●	Shape
	●	Normal angles (see below)
Position	●	Normal articulations
	●	No valgus or varus deformity (relation to talus and cuboid)
Structure	●	Mineralization
	●	Normal trabeculation
	●	Sharp delineation of trabecular pattern
	●	No circumscribed or diffuse densities or decalcified areas (e.g., bandlike, patchy, cystic)
Contours	●	Cortex smooth, sharp, and of normal thickness (no circumscribed thickening or thinning)
	●	No contour defects or discontinuities
	●	No bony excrescences or calcifications (especially involving the Achilles' tendon or plantar aponeurosis)
	●	No periosteal reaction
Joint	●	Shape of articular surfaces (congruent)
	●	Contours (smooth, sharp)
	●	Joint space
	●	No intra-articular or periarticular calcifications
	●	Accessory bones at typical location
Soft tissues	●	Intact
	●	Normal thickness (soft-tissue shadow of heel, see below)
	●	No foreign bodies

Important Data

1. *Angle between the calcaneal tuberosity and subtalar joint line* = 30–40°
2. *Angle of calcaneal axis* = ca. 15°
3. *Soft-tissue shadow of heel:* up to 25 mm thick in men or 23 mm in women

Tarsus, Biplane Views

The individual tarsal and metatarsal bones are normal in shape, size, number, and position. They show proper mineralization and bone structure.

The cortical borders are smooth, sharply delineated, and of normal thickness with no abnormal contour defects.

The tarsal articular surfaces are normally shaped, smooth, and sharply marginated. All the joint spaces are of normal width.

The soft tissues are unremarkable.

Interpretation

The tarsus appears normal.

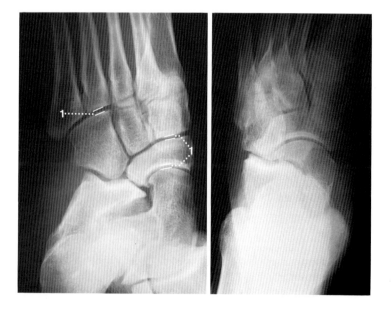

Checklist

Shape	• Number:
	— Navicular bone (consists of one part)
	— Cuboid bone
	— Three cuneiform bones (medial, intermediate, lateral)
	— First through fifth metatarsals
	— Distal portions of talus and calcaneus
	• Shape
	• Size
Position	• Interrelationship of the tarsal bones
Structure	• Mineralization
	• Normal trabeculation
	• Sharp delineation of the trabecular pattern
	• No circumscribed lucencies (cystic, bandlike, patchy, diffuse; e.g., navicular bone in aseptic necrosis or medial cuneiform bone in osteochondronecrosis) (Caution: the lateral half of the cuboid bone normally appears hyperlucent.)
	• No abnormal densities
Contours	• Cortex smooth and sharp
	• Normal cortical thickness
	• No contour defects, impressions, or discontinuities
	• No subchondral sclerosis or erosions
	• No marginal osteophytes
	• No bony excrescences (e.g., on the cuneiform bone)
Joints	• Shape of joints
	• Normal width of joint spaces (see below)
	• Accessory bones at typical location (with normal bone structure and intact cortex) (e.g., os tibiale externum between navicular bone and head of talus)
	• No intra-articular or periarticular calcifications
Soft tissues	• No swelling, no foreign bodies
	• No calcifications (vascular or at tendon attachments)

Important Data

1. *Width of joint spaces* = 2–2.5 mm (intertarsal, metatarsal, and tarsometatarsal joints)

Forefoot, Biplane Views

The pedal skeleton is normal in the shape, size, and number of the phalanges, metatarsals, and visible tarsal bones. The position of the phalanges is normal in relation to the metatarsals.

Mineralization and bone structure are normal. The cortex is smooth, sharply defined, and of normal thickness with no pathological contour defects.

The articular surfaces are normally shaped, smooth, and sharply marginated and are separated by joint spaces of normal width. There are no intra-articular or periarticular calcifications.

The soft tissues are unremarkable.

Interpretation

The bones and soft tissues of the forefoot appear normal.

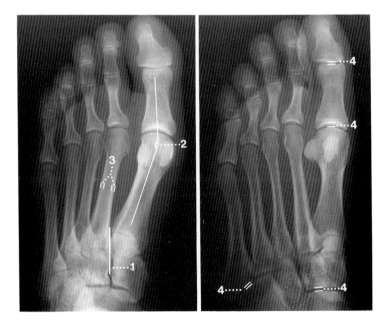

Checklist

Shape	•	Number (5 rays; 5 metatarsals; 5 proximal, middle, and distal phalanges; 3 cuneiform bones; cuboid bone)
	•	Size
Position	•	Normal interrelationship of the metatarsals and phalanges
	•	No separation of the metatarsal heads
	•	Proximal phalanx of big toe (see below)
	•	No subluxation of the second metatarsal (see below)
Structure	•	Mineralization
	•	Trabeculation
	•	Sharp delineation of the trabecular pattern
	•	No circumscribed lucencies or densities (especially in the head of the second metatarsal, as in type II Köhler disease = aseptic necrosis)
	•	Harmonious width of medullary cavities
	•	Epiphyseal plates (open/closed)
Contours	•	Cortex smooth and sharp
	•	Normal cortical bone thickness (see below)
	•	No contour defects or discontinuities
	•	No periosteal reaction or elevation
	•	No sclerosis
	•	Intact subchondral plate
Joint	•	Normal width of joint spaces (see below)
	•	No marginal osteophytes
	•	No subchondral sclerosis or erosions
	•	Accessory bones at typical location
	•	No intra-articular or periarticular calcifications
Soft tissues	•	Normal thickness
	•	No foreign bodies
	•	Fat planes apposed to the bone (especially near joints)
	•	No calcifications (vascular or at tendon attachments)

Important Data

1. *Subluxation line* without a stepoff (second metatarsal)
2. *Valgus angle of big toe:* <20° = normal
3. *Total cortical bone thickness* (midshaft, second metatarsal) = ca. 5 mm
4. *Width of joint spaces* = 2–2.5 mm (intertarsal, metatarsal, and tarsometatarsal joints)

Toe, Biplane Views

The phalanges are of normal shape (including the distal phalanx, within the range of variation) and show proper position and alignment. Mineralization and bone structure are normal. The cortical borders are smooth and sharp with no abnormal contour defects. Cortical thickness is normal. The lanula is intact.

The proximal and distal articular surfaces have an anatomically normal shape and smooth margins. The joint spaces are of normal width throughout. There are no intra-articular or periarticular calcifications. The soft tissues are unremarkable.

Interpretation

The toe appears normal.

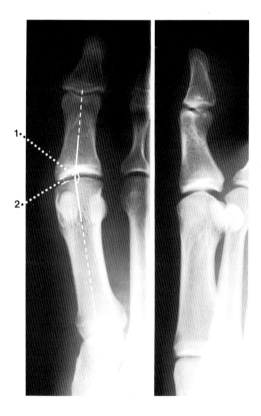

Checklist

Shape	•	Number (metatarsal bone plus proximal, and distal phalanges)
	•	Shape
Position	•	Straight axial alignment (no lateral deviation)
Structure	•	Mineralization
	•	Trabeculation
	•	Sharp delineation of the trabecular pattern
	•	No circumscribed lucencies or densities
	•	Harmonious width of the medullary cavities
	•	Epiphyseal plates (open/closed)
Contours	•	Cortex smooth and sharp
	•	Normal cortical bone thickness
	•	No contour defects or discontinuities
	•	No periosteal reaction or elevation
	•	No sclerosis
	•	No cortical bone dissections
Joints	•	Shape (congruent)
	•	Articular surfaces (smooth, sharp)
	•	No cysts or erosions
	•	No marginal osteophytes
	•	Width of joint spaces (see below)
	•	No intra-articular or periarticular calcifications
	•	No isolated bone fragments
	•	Accessory bones at typical location
Soft tissues	•	Intact
	•	Normal thickness
	•	No calcifications (vascular or at tendon attachments)

Important Data

1. *Valgus angle of big toe:* <20° = normal
2. *Width of joint spaces* = 1–2 mm

Stress Radiographs

Stress Radiographs of the Knee

With the knee clamped in a flexed position, a force of approximately 15 kp is applied to the selected aspect of the knee joint or to the upper tibia.

The films demonstrate normal relative positions of the femoral and tibial articular surfaces under loading. The articular surfaces and joint spaces conform to the nonstress views.

Interpretation

The stressed knee joint appears normal, with no radiographic evidence of a ligamentous lesion.

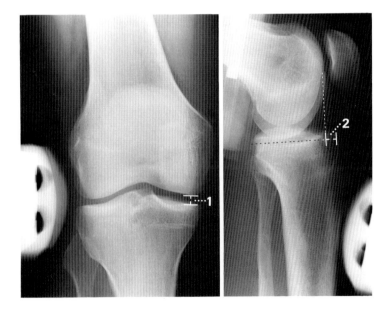

Checklist

Procedure	•	1. The knee is clamped in a holding device (or held manually) in a position of 20° flexion A pressure of 15 kp (25 kp) is applied to the medial or lateral side of the knee joint. AP radiographs are obtained (to test collateral ligament stability)
	•	2. The knee is clamped in a holding device (or held manually) in a position of 90° flexion A pressure of 15 kp (25 kp) is applied to the patella or 2 cm below the tibial plateau (or the examiner pulls the upper tibia forward or pushes it backward with both hands). Lateral radiographs are taken of both knees (pulling tests the anterior cruciate ligament, pushing tests the posterior cruciate ligament)
Knee joint	•	Test 1 should show normal medial or posterior opening of the joint space (see below)
	•	Test 2 should show no increase in anterior or posterior drawer mobility compared with the opposite side
Contours	•	No contour defects or discontinuities (change relative to nonstress views?)
	•	No intra-articular loose bodies

Important Data

1. *Medial or lateral opening of the joint space:*
   - Less than 5 mm = normal
   - Between 5 and 10 mm = equivocal (compare with opposite side: >3 mm discrepancy is abnormal)
   - More than 10 mm = abnormal (should still be compared with opposite side)
2. *Drawer sign* (anterior or posterior displacement of upper tibia): >3 mm more than the opposite side = abnormal (should still be compared with opposite side)

Stress Radiographs of the Ankle Joint

With the foot clamped in a holding device, a force of approximately 15 kp is applied above the lateral or medial malleolus with the foot internally rotated, and an equal force is applied to the distal anterior tibial margin with the knee in 30° flexion. Stress radiographs of the ankle joint are then obtained in the AP and lateral projections.

The aperture angle between the tibia and talus within normal limits on the medial and lateral sides. Talar advancement is normal.

The articular surfaces and joint spaces conforms to the nonstress views.

Interpretation

The stressed ankle joint appears normal, with no excessive lateral or medial opening of the joint space and normal talar advancement. There is no radiographic evidence of a ligamentous lesion.

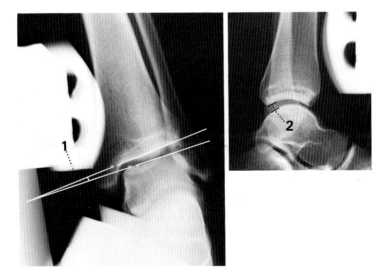

Checklist

Procedure
- 1. The foot is clamped in a holding device (or held manually) in a position of internal rotation
A pressure of 15 kp is applied above the medial or lateral malleolus.
AP radiographs are obtained
- 2. The foot is clamped in a holding device (or held manually) with the knee flexed 30°
A pressure of 15 kp is applied to the distal anterior tibial margin
Lateral radiographs are obtained

Ankle joint
- Test 1 should demonstrate a normal aperture angle between the tibia and talus (see below)
- Test 2 should demonstrate normal talar advancement (see below)

Contours
- No contour defects or discontinuities (change relative to nonstress views?)
- No intra-articular loose bodies

Important Data

1. *Aperture angle between the tibia and talus*(medial and lateral):
   - Less than 5° = normal
   - Between 5° and 10° = equivocal (compare with opposite side: <3° discrepancy is normal, >3° is abnormal)
   - More than 10° = abnormal (may require comparison with opposite side)
2. *Talar advancement:*
   - Less than 5 mm = normal
   - Between 5 and 10 mm = equivocal (compare with opposite side: <3 mm discrepancy is normal, >3 mm is abnormal)
   - More than 10 mm = abnormal (may require comparison with opposite side)

Other Plain Films

Chest, Biplane Views

The diaphragm has smooth contours, a normal arched shape, and occupies a normal position. The costophrenic angles are clear. Both lungs are normally aerated and are applied to the chest wall on all sides. Pulmonary structure is normal and shows normal vascular markings.

The mediastinum is centered and of normal width. The trachea shows a normal position, borders, and diameter with no thickening of the paratracheal lines. The cardiac and vascular shadows show a normal configuration. The thoracic skeleton is symmetrically shaped, and the thoracic spine is unremarkable.

The soft-tissue envelope of the chest shows no abnormalities.

Interpretation

The lungs and heart appear normal.

Checklist

Diaphragm	• Position (ca. 10th–11th posterior ribs)
	• Sharp costophrenic angle
	• No effusion or adhesions
Pleural space	• Lung applied to the chest wall on all sides
	• No circumscribed pleural thickening
	• No calcifications
Pulmonary structure	• Symmetrical radiolucency (scoliosis, projection!)
	• Clear and aerated (no infiltrates, focal densities, calcific structures, Kerley lines)
Pulmonary vessels	• Caliber (see below)
	• No pruning of peripheral vessels
	• Course

Mediastinum	• Shape, size, position (centered)
	• Normal radiographic density (no abnormal lucencies)
	• Trachea centered (lumen—see below; smooth contours, not narrowed by a goiter or other mass)
	• Pleural contact lines not displaced (paravertebral, paratracheal, anterior and posterior pleural contact lines)
Hilum	• Shape, width (mass lesion?), position, calcifications
Heart	• Size (see below)
	• Configuration (normal, aortic, mitral with normal inspiration)
	• Normal cardiac waist (left atrial appendage, pulmonary segment; no fullness of upper left cardiac border)
	• *Left ventricle:* caval triangle intact
	• *Right ventricle:* no thickening of retrosternal contact surface
	• *Left atrium:* atrial shadow not accentuated, acute angle of carina (see below), no narrowing of upper retrocardiac space
	• *Right atrium:* no right-sided cardiac prominence (AP view)
	• *Aortic arch:* configuration (no elongation, calcification), position (descends slightly to left of midline)
Bony thorax	• Symmetry
	• Ribs: shape, position, contours (smooth, no defects), structure
	• Thoracic spine: position, shape, contours (degenerative changes?)
	• Clavicle, components of shoulder joint
Soft tissues	• Swelling?
	• Foreign bodies?
	• Calcifications?
	• Emphysema?

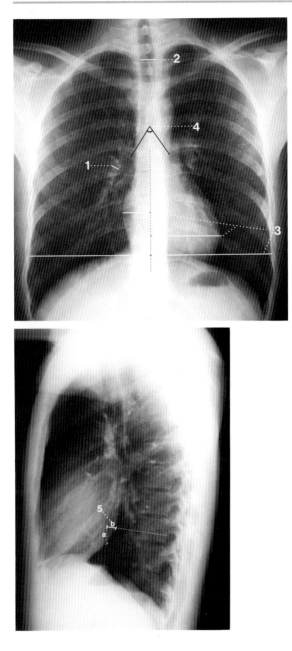

Important Data

1. *Caliber of pulmonary vessels:*
   Right pulmonary artery: up to 14 mm in women, up to 16 mm in men; >17 mm is definitely abnormal (measured at origin of intermediate bronchus)
2. *Tracheal lumen* = ca. 1.5 cm
3. *Cardiac size:* ratio of transverse diameters of heart and lung = 1:2
4. *Tracheal bifurcation angle* = ca. 55–65°
5. *Caval triangle:* b < 18 mm = normal
   (a = 2 cm [course of vena cava], b = parallel to vertebral body endplate)

Chest, Right Anterior Oblique View (First Oblique Diameter, Fencer Position)

The diaphragm is normally positioned and has smooth margins. The costophrenic angle is clear. Both lungs are fully expanded, and the visible portions show normal pulmonary structure with no infiltrates or nodular densities.

The heart has a normal configuration. The right atrium, left ventricle, pulmonary outflow tract, and especially the ascending aorta are of normal size. The pulmonary vessels are normal.

Imaged portions of the thoracic skeleton are unremarkable.

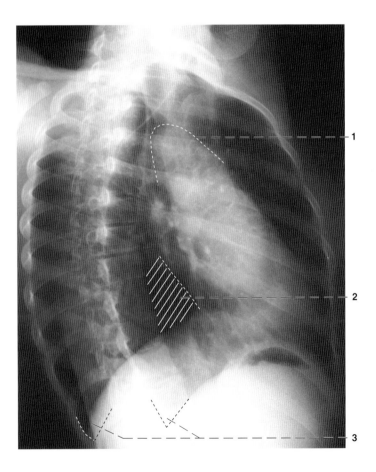

Interpretation

The heart and lungs appear normal.

Checklist

Diaphragm	• Position (ca. 10th–11th posterior ribs)
	• Sharp costophrenic angle, not obscured by effusion or adhesions **(3)**
Pleural space	• Lung applied to the chest wall on all sides
	• No circumscribed pleural thickening
	• No calcifications
Pulmonary structure	• No infiltrates or nodules, normal fine structure (especially the posterolateral right lung and anterolateral left lung)
Pulmonary vessels	• Caliber (especially the inferior pulmonary veins on the left side)
Mediastinum	• Shape, size, position
	• Esophagus (if opacified) should descend in an almost straight, posterosuperior-to-anteroinferior course (sensitive indicator of cardiac enlargement)
Heart	• Size, configuration; best displayed are the left atrium, the anterosuperior part of the left ventricle, the conus arteriosus, and the pulmonary outflow tract (pulmonary trunk)
	• Ascending aorta (the descending aorta is less clearly portrayed) and aortic arch (caliber, no elongation, calcification) **(1)**
	• Left ventricle: caval triangle intact **(2)**
Thoracic skeleton	• Ribs: shape, position, contours (smooth, no defects), structure
	• Thoracic spine: position, bone structure, vertebral body height, disk space height, apophyseal joints
Soft tissues	• Swelling, foreign bodies, calcifications, emphysema?

Chest, Left Anterior Oblique View (Second Oblique Diameter, Boxer Position)

The diaphragm is orthotopic with smooth margins, and the costophrenic angle is clear. Both lungs are fully expanded. Evaluable lung zones display normal pulmonary structure with no infiltrates or nodular densities. The trachea and tracheal bifurcation are unremarkable.

The heart has a normal configuration. The ventricles, ascending aorta, and aortic arch are of normal size. There are no abnormal calcifications projected over the cardiac valves.

The large pulmonary vessels appear normal.

Imaged portions of the thoracic skeleton are unremarkable.

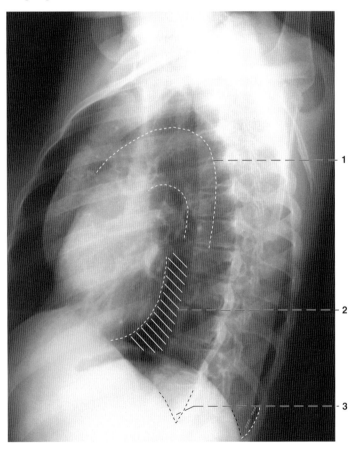

Interpretation

The heart and lungs appear normal.

Checklist

Diaphragm	• Position (ca. 10th–11th posterior ribs)
	• Sharp costophrenic angle, not obscured by effusion or adhesions **(3)**
Pleural space	• Lung applied to the chest wall on all sides
	• No circumscribed pleural thickening
	• No calcifications
Pulmonary structure	• The anterolateral right lung and posterolateral left lung are most clearly visualized
	• No infiltrates or nodules, normal fine structure
Pulmonary vessels	• Caliber (especially the pulmonary arteries and the inferior pulmonary veins on the left side)
Mediastinum	• Shape, size, position
	• Trachea and tracheal bifurcation
	• Esophagus (if opacified) should descend in an almost straight, posterosuperior-to-anteroinferior course (sensitive indicator of cardiac enlargement)
Heart	• Size, configuration; best displayed are the anterior border of the right ventricle and the posteroinferior border of the left ventricle **(2)**
	• Cardiac valves: Aortic valve (note: the aorta should appear to arise from the center of the heart) *Pulmonary valve* (note: the highest of the cardiac valves) *Tricuspid valve* (right atrium/ventricle) *Mitral valve* (left atrium/ventricle)
	• Ascending aorta, aortic arch (which appears "unwound" in this projection: caliber, no elongation, calcification **[1]**), descending aorta
Thoracic skeleton	• Ribs: shape, position, contours (smooth, no defects), structure
	• Thoracic spine: position, bone structure, vertebral body height, disk space height, apophyseal joints
Soft tissues	• Swelling, foreign bodies, calcifications, emphysema?

Upright Abdomen

The diaphragm has sharp borders, a normal arched shape, and occupies a normal position. There is no evidence of free air below the diaphragmatic leaflets. The air-filled portions of the gastrointestinal tract appear normal and show a normal gas distribution. There are no distended bowel loops or fluid levels.

The soft-tissue shadows of the liver, spleen, kidneys, and bladder are unremarkable. There are no abnormal calcifications or radiopaque foreign bodies projected over the abdomen.

Muscle and soft-tissue shadows appear normal.

Imaged skeletal structures are unremarkable.

Interpretation

The abdomen appears normal.

Checklist

Diaphragm	• Shape (domelike convexity of leaflets)
	• Position (see below)
	• Contours (smooth, sharp)
	• No free air below the diaphragm leaflets (gastric bubble!)
Gastrointes- tinal tract	• Normal gas distribution (stomach, small and large intestine)
	• No distended bowel segments, fluid levels, or standing loops
	• No displacement of bowel segments
	• Normal colonic haustrations
	• Bowel wall (thickness, air inclusions? contours: thumbprinting?)
Liver, spleen	• Shape
	• Size (see below)
	• Contours of inferior splenic and hepatic borders (smooth, sharp)
	• Position
	• Structure: homogeneous, no calcifications, no air (e.g., in the bile ducts)
Kidneys (bladder)	• Shape
	• Size (if evaluable)
	• Position (see below), axis (superiorly convergent)
	• Calculi? (including the urinary drainage tract)
Soft tissues	• No soft-tissue masses
	• No calcifications (e.g., pancreas, ovaries, uterus, kidneys, ureters, bladder, vessels)
	• No foreign bodies
	• Muscle planes and shadows (if visualized)
	• Gas in the organs?
	• Normal flank markings (see below)
Skeleton	• Shape
	• Position
	• Structure (vertebral arches intact, no lucencies or densities)
	• Contours (intact, smooth, no osteophytes)

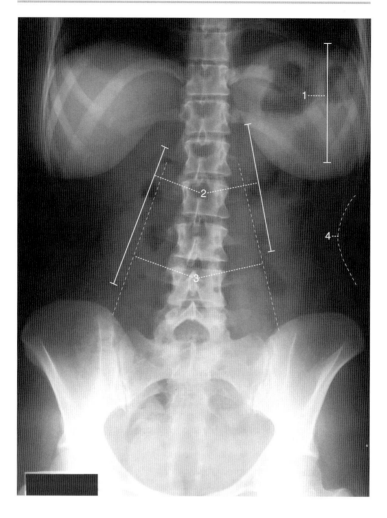

Important Data

Position of diaphragm: ca. 10th–11th posterior ribs
1. *Splenic size:* up to 15 cm between left hemidiaphragm and lower pole of spleen
2. *Renal position:* ca. from L1 to L4 (right kidney is 2 cm lower) Kidneys are approx. 1.5 vertebral bodies lower than in the supine view
   Renal axes converge superiorly

Muscle planes:
3. Psoas

Flank markings:
4. Preperitoneal fat
   Abdominal musculature (if visualized)
   Subcutaneous fat (if visualized)

Supine Abdomen

The visualized soft tissues show no abnormalities. There is no sign of calcifications or radiopaque foreign bodies. The air-filled portions of the gastrointestinal tract appear normal and show a normal gas distribution.

The soft-tissue shadows of the liver, spleen, kidneys, and bladder are unremarkable and indicate normal organ sizes and positions.

The muscle shadows have smooth, sharp margins. Flank markings are normal.

Imaged skeletal structures are unremarkable.

Interpretation

The abdomen appears normal.

Checklist

Soft tissues	• No soft-tissue masses
	• No calcifications (e.g., pancreas, ovaries, uterus, kidneys, ureters, bladder, vessels)
	• No foreign bodies
	• Muscle planes and shadows (not obliterated, see below)
	• Gas projected onto organs?
	• Normal flank markings (see below)
Gastrointestinal tract	• Normal gas distribution (stomach, small and large intestine)
	• No distended bowel segments, no "football sign"
	• No displacement of bowel segments
	• Normal colonic haustrations
	• Bowel wall (thickness, air inclusions?)
Diaphragm	• Shape, contours (if visualized)
Liver, spleen	• Shape
	• Size
	• Contours of inferior splenic and hepatic borders (smooth, sharp)
	• Position
	• Structure: homogeneous, no calcifications, no air (e.g., in the bile ducts)
Kidneys, bladder	• Shape
	• Size (see below)
	• Position (see below)
	• Axis (superiorly convergent, see below)
	• No calculi (including the urinary drainage tract)
	• Normal density of suprarenal fat triangle (adrenals)
Skeleton	• Shape
	• Position
	• Structure (no lucencies or densities)
	• Contours (intact, smooth, no osteophytes)
	• Vertebral arches intact

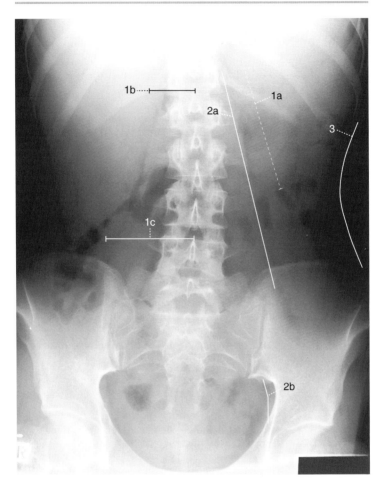

Important Data

1. *Kidneys*
   (**a**) Size: ca. 13 cm × 6 cm ($\leq$ 2 cm difference between right and left kidneys)
   Position: approx. from T12 to L3 (right kidney 2 cm lower)
   Renal axes converge superiorly:
   (**b**) Distance from superior pole to center of spinal column: 4–5 cm
   (**c**) Distance from inferior pole to center of spinal column: 6–9 cm
2. *Muscle planes*
   (**a**) Psoas
   (**b**) Obturator internus
3. *Flank markings* (from deep to superficial): preperitoneal fat, abdominal musculature, subcutaneous fat

Spot Film Radiography

Biplane Mammograms

The breasts are normally shaped and reasonably symmetrical. There are no discrete palpable masses or other palpable abnormalities.

The mammograms show normal development of the breast parenchyma with normal radiographic density and a homogeneous fine structure. There are no circumscribed soft-tissue densities or calcifications, and there is no abnormal increase in connective tissue permeation. The skin and subcutaneous tissues are of normal thickness.

Interpretation

Both breasts appear normal, with no evidence of malignancy.

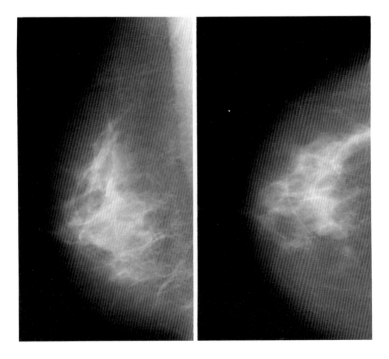

Checklist

Inspection and palpation	• Size
	• Shape
	• Symmetry
	• Consistency
	• No circumscribed firmness
	• No dimpling of the skin
	• No nipple retraction
	• No fixation of the glandular tissue
	• No expressible nipple discharge
	• No lymph node enlargement

Mammographic findings:

Breast parenchyma and fat	• Size (proportion of breast parenchyma to fat)
	• Involuted breast parenchyma (shape, symmetry, normal septation by fatty tissue)
	• Uniform fine structure
	• Density of individual parenchymal areas
	• Extent of connective tissue permeation
	• No discrete soft-tissue densities
	• No spiculated densities
	• No calcifications (clustered microcalcifications; intraductal, lobular, ringlike, disseminated calcifications)
	• Vessels (calcific deposits?)
Axilla	• Homogeneous density
	• No circumscribed soft-tissue densities consistent with enlarged lymph nodes
Skin	• Skin thickness (viewed tangentially, no circumscribed thickening)
	• No dimpling
	• No circumscribed densities in the subcutaneous tissue

Tracheal Spot Film

The trachea is normally positioned, appearing as a lucent band. The pharynx and trachea are of normal shape and diameter. Their inner walls are smooth and sharp. The laryngeal cartilages and hyoid bone are normal in shape and position. The vocal cords are normally developed and display normal function.

The imaged skeletal structures and cervical soft tissues are unremarkable, with a normal width of the retropharyngeal and retrotracheal spaces.

Interpretation

The trachea appears normal.

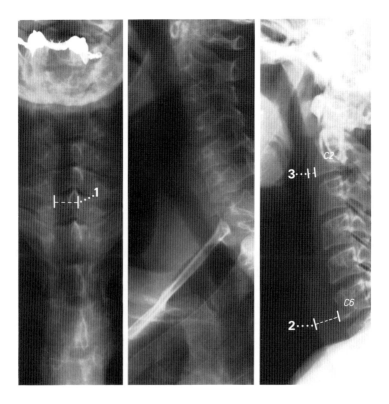

Checklist

Position	• Central (with a normal position of the cervical and thoracic spine)
Shape	• Pharynx (nasopharynx, oropharynx, hypopharynx)
	• Trachea (diameter, see below)
	• No abnormal impressions (aortic impression is normal)
	• No narrowing or expansion
	• No densities or radiopaque foreign bodies
	• Bifurcation angle (if visualized, see below)
Contours	• Smooth and sharp, no discontinuities
	• Normal wall thickness
	• Tracheal cartilages (borders, density)
Larynx	• Shape (symmetry)
	• Position (see below)
	• Smooth, sharp contours
	• Vocal cords (shape, function: I and U phonation, forced expiration)
Soft tissues	• Soft-tissue envelope intact, no swelling
	• No abnormal calcifications or foreign bodies
	• Normal width of retrotracheal and retropharyngeal spaces (see below)
	• No widening of the prevertebral soft-tissue shadow
Skeleton	• Shape
	• Position (axial alignment)
	• Structure
	• Contours

Important Data

1. Tracheal diameter = 15–23.5 mm in men, 11.5–18 mm in women
2. Width of retrotracheal space = 8–22 mm in adults (measured at C6 level)
   Bifurcation angle = 55–65°
   Position of hyoid bone = ca. C3–C4 level
   Position of cricoid cartilage = ca. C5–C6 level
3. Width of retropharyngeal space = up to 7 mm in adults (at C2 level) (check for accurate lateral projection!)

Conventional Tomography

Tomography of the Pulmonary Hilum

The normal tracheal bifurcation and the primary divisions of the two main bronchi were imaged by linear tomography in 10 sections acquired at 1-cm intervals in the AP projection.

The trachea appears as a central lucent band with a normal diameter and smooth contours. The main bronchi arise normally at the tracheal bifurcation and divide normally into lobar and segmental bronchi. All imaged segments of the tracheobronchial system show a clear lumen of normal diameter with normal-appearing bronchial walls. There are no abnormal densities in the course of the bronchi. The pulmonary vessels are unremarkable.

Imaged portions of the lung display normal pulmonary structure. The visualized portions of the aorta, vena cava, and heart show no abnormalities.

Interpretation

The pulmonary hilar region appears normal. In particular, there is no evidence of a mass lesion and no narrowing of the tracheobronchial system.

Checklist

Technique
- Tomographic motion (linear, circular, elliptical, spiral, etc.)
- Spacing of the sections (usually 1 cm for the hilum)
- Number of sections required
- Coverage

Trachea
- Position (central, not displaced)
- Diameter (see below)
- Contours: smooth and sharp, no discontinuities
- Wall thickness (no circumscribed change, no calcifications)
- Tracheal cartilages
- Tracheal bifurcation (angle, see below)

Right main bronchus	•	Angle of origin
	•	Diameter (see below)
	•	Division:

— Upper lobe bronchus (OL): segment 1 (apical), 2 (posterior), 3 (anterior)
— *Intermediate bronchus* (Bi): parallel to right pulmonary artery
— *Middle lobe bronchus* (ML): segment 4 (lateral), 5 (medial)
— *Lower lobe bronchus* (UL): segment 6 (apical or superior), 7 (mediobasal or cardial), 8 (anterobasal), 9 (laterobasal), 10 (posterobasal)

Left main bronchus	•	*Upper lobe bronchus* (OL): segment 1/2 (apicoposterior), 3 (anterior)

— Lingula (Li): 4 (superior), 5 (inferior)
— Lower lobe bronchus (UL): segment 6 (apical), 7/8 (anterobasal), 9 (laterobasal), 10 (posterobasal)
— Bronchi:
  Patent, no stenosis or occlusion
  Caliber (no narrowing or dilatation)
  No abrupt caliber changes
  Smooth walls, no discontinuities
  Normal wall thickness
  No bronchial masses of soft-tissue or calcific density
  Course (no displacement, splaying, or bunching)
— Pulmonary vessels
  Course (arteries follow bronchi, veins are more horizontal)
  Caliber (see below), no abrupt changes

Other structures	•	*Pulmonary structure* is normal

No opacities (soft-tissue, calcific)
Normal lobar boundaries

• *Aorta:*
— Normal diameter, no elongation or displacement
— No calcifications
• *Heart:* size (if evaluable), calcifications?

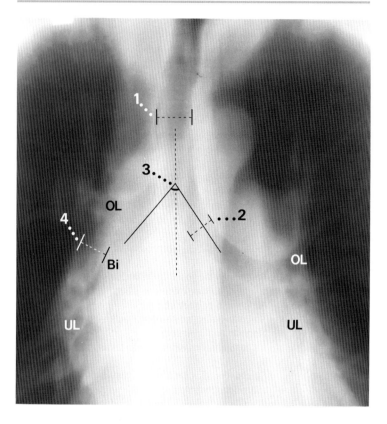

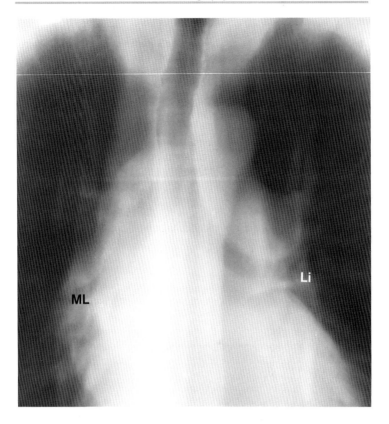

Important Data

1. *Tracheal lumen* = 11–18 mm in women, 15–23 mm in men
2. *Diameters of main bronchi* = right ca. 15 mm, left ca. 13 mm
3. *Carinal angle* = ca. 55–65°
4. *Caliber of pulmonary vessels:*
   Right pulmonary artery = up to 14 mm in women, up to 16 mm in men; >17 mm is definitely abnormal (measured at origin of intermediate bronchus)

AP Tomography of the Sacroiliac Joints

The sacroiliac joints were imaged by linear tomography in 10 sections acquired at 10-mm intervals in the AP projection.

The articular surfaces display a normal, symmetrical shape on all sections. The cortical borders are smooth and sharp with no abnormal contour defects, and cortical thickness is normal. The subchondral areas are unremarkable. The joint space is of normal width on all sections. There are no intra-articular loose bodies.

Imaged portions of the ilium and sacrum are anatomically normal and symmetrical, showing proper mineralization and bone structure.

The soft tissues visible in the imaged planes show no abnormalities.

Interpretation

The sacroiliac joints have a normal tomographic appearance.

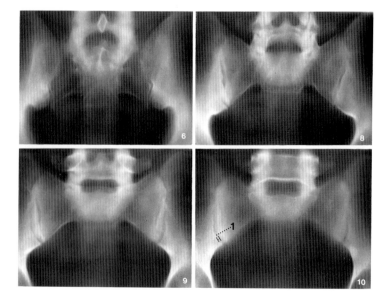

Checklist

Technique	• Tomographic motion (linear, circular, elliptical, spiral, etc.)
	• Spacing of the sections (usually 1 cm for the sacroiliac joint)
	• Number of sections required
	• Coverage

Joint:

Shape	• Articular surfaces converge superiorly
	• Symmetrical (accurate projections?)
Contours	• Cortex smooth and sharp, normal cortical thickness
	• No contour defects or discontinuities
	• No bandlike, patchy, or circumscribed densities
	• No erosive or destructive changes, no cysts
	• No sclerosis
	• Symmetry
Joint	• Normal width of joint space (see below)
	• No circumscribed widening
	• No ankylosis
	• No lucencies (air)
	• Symmetry

Bone:

Shape	• Sacrum (4 pairs of foramina, 5 vertebrae); symmetrical
	• Mineralization
	• Sharp delineation of the trabecular pattern (including subchondral bone)
	• No circumscribed lucencies or densities
Soft tissues	• No calcifications in ligaments, tendons, or fasciae
	• No radiopaque foreign bodies or calcifications (lymph nodes, vessels)

Important Data

1. *Width of sternoclavicular joint space* = 3–5 mm

Contrast Examinations Gastrointestinal Tract

Esophagus

The esophagus is centrally positioned and transmits the swallowed contrast bolus normally and without obstruction. Esophageal motility is normal, and all segments show normal distenion with no intraluminal filling defects.

The wall is smoothly contoured and shows a delicate, predominantly longitudinal rugal pattern.

Contrast medium passes unobstructed from the esophagus into the stomach, with no evidence of a hiatal hernia or excessive gastroesophageal reflux.

Imaged portions of the neck and thorax are unremarkable.

Interpretation

The esophagus appears normal by esophagography.

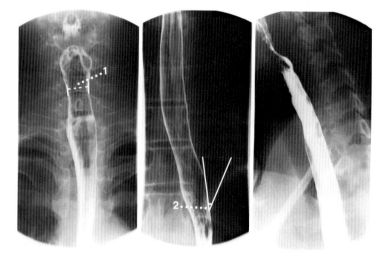

Checklist

Preliminary fluoroscopy	• No radiopaque foreign bodies
	• No soft-tissue swelling (e.g., goiter)
	• Tracheal air column is centered
Position, motility, shape	• Esophagus is approximately centered (e.g., not displaced by a goiter)
	• Deglutition (the epiglottis completely seals the trachea)
	• Transit is not delayed (see below) or obstructed
	• All wall segments show equal distensibility (except at physiological constrictions: aorta, trachea, hiatus)
	• No sites of fixed luminal narrowing or dilatation
	• No filling defects (e.g., intraluminal foreign bodies)
Contours	• Smooth and sharp
	• Delicate, predominantly longitudinal pattern of mucosal folds
	• No cutoff of folds, no contrast pooling
	• No convergence of folds, no persistent niche
	• No hernia-like outpouchings
	• No garland-like protrusions (varices occur mainly in the distal esophagus) during a Valsalva maneuver
Esophageal emptying	• Not delayed or obstructed
	• Normal esophagogastric angle (see below)
	• No excessive gastroesophageal reflux
	• No hiatal hernia (axial sliding hernia, paraesophageal hernia) (may use provocative test with head-down tilt)
Surrounding structures	• Skeleton (shape, position; e.g., scoliosis, vertebral body spurs)
	• Tracheal wall, main bronchi (shape, position, diameter)
	• Cervical soft tissues
	• Heart (left atrium, left ventricle, especially in lateral view)
	• No extraluminal foreign bodies

Important Data

Esophageal transit time: ca. 3 seconds with a small bolus
1. *Luminal diameter of the esophagus:* 9–13 mm (at cricoid level)
2. *Esophagogastric angle:* ca. 85–90°

Stomach and Duodenum

Deglutition is normal. The esophagus is unremarkable, showing a normal luminal diameter and smooth contours. Contrast medium passes unobstructed from the esophagus into the stomach, with no evidence of a hiatal hernia or excessive gastroesophageal reflux.

The stomach presents a normal shape, smooth contours, and a normal mucosal pattern. All gastric segments show normal distensibility, and contrast transit is unimpaired. The pylorus opens centrally into the duodenal bulb.

The duodenal bulb shows good distensibility. As in the stomach, there is a normal rugal pattern with no pooling of retained contrast medium. The duodenal sweep shows no splaying, mass lesions, inflammatory changes, or other abnormalities.

Interpretation

The stomach and duodenum appear normal.

Checklist

Preliminary fluoroscopy	• No extraintestinal or intraperitoneal air
	• No air–fluid levels
	• No radiopaque foreign bodies
Techniques	• (a) Full-column study
	• (b) Double-contrast study
	• (c) Double-contrast hypotonic study
Esophagus	• Deglutition (transit not delayed or obstructed, see below)
	• Luminal diameter (see below) and distensibility
	• Contours (smooth contours, fine mucosal relief)
	• Esophageal emptying (unobstructed, normal esophagogastric angle—see below)
	— No hiatal hernia or gastroesophageal reflux (provocative test with head-down tilt)
Stomach	• Shape:
	— J shape, fishhook, cascade, steerhorn, transverse
	• Contours:
	— Smooth outer contours
	— Normal, intricate (not coarsened), continuous rugal pattern and fine mucosal relief (double-contrast study)
	— No pooling of contrast material
	— No filling defect, niche, or convergence of mucosal folds
	— No mass impression
Duodenal bulb	• Centered pyloric orifice
	• Unobstructed contrast transit
	• Uniform, unimpaired distensibility
	• No fold convergence, niche, or contrast pooling
Duodenal sweep	• Shape (no splaying of duodenal C loop)
	• No mass impression or constriction
	• No filling defect or persistent niche
	• No outpouchings or protrusions (especially on the inner aspect of the duodenal sweep)

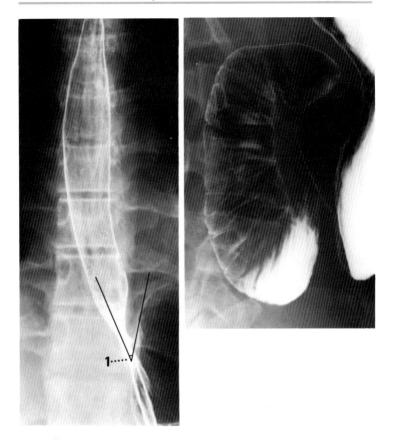

Important Data

Esophageal transit time: ca. 3 seconds
Luminal diameter of the esophagus: 9–13 mm (at the cricoid level)
1. *Esophagogastric angle:* ca. 85–90°

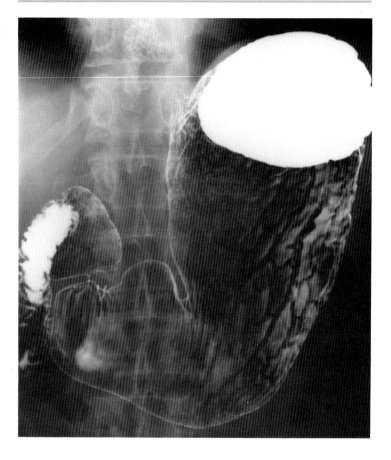

Upper Gastrointestinal Series

See Stomach and Duodenum.
There is normal transit through the jejunum and ileum. Individual loops of small intestine show no abnormalities. The terminal ileum is properly shaped and terminates normally in the lower pole of the cecum.

Interpretation

The upper GI series appear normal.

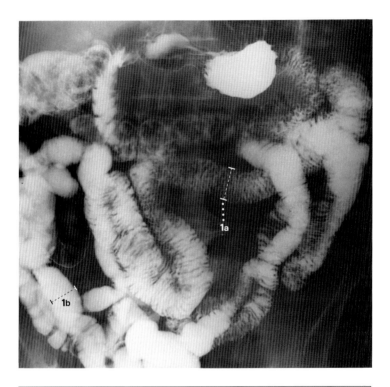

Important Data

1. (**a**) Jejunal lumen: approx. 3 cm
   (**b**) Ileal lumen: smaller than the jejunum

Checklist

Same as under Stomach and Duodenum

Small intestine	• No delay of transit through the jejunum and ileum
	• Fine feathery rugal pattern in the jejunum
	• No haustration of the ileal mucosa
	• Normal luminal diameters (see Important Data)
	• No dilatation or stenosis
	• No segmental motility disorder
	• No fixation of individual bowel loops (freely displaceable on palpation)
	• Clear projection of bowel loops
Ileocecal region	• Terminal ileum opens into lower pole of cecum (arrow)
	• Unobstructed contrast transit across ileocecal junction
	• Normal lumen compared with rest of ileum
	• No constriction
	• No fistulation
	• No mass effects
	• Preservation of normal mucosal relief

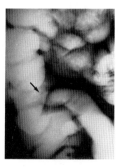

Small Bowel Enema (Enteroclysis)

Following partial anesthesia of the nasopharynx, the enteroclysis tube is introduced perorally. The tube is positioned distal to the ligament of Treitz, and ca. 160 mL contrast medium and 1.5 L methylcellulose are instilled.

The small-bowel loops in this study show normal distensibility, a normal course, and normal luminal diameters. All palpable small-bowel loops show normal motility and deformability. The wall contours are smooth and show a normal fold pattern. The terminal ileum and ileocecal junction are unremarkable.

Interpretation

The jejunum and ileum appear normal.

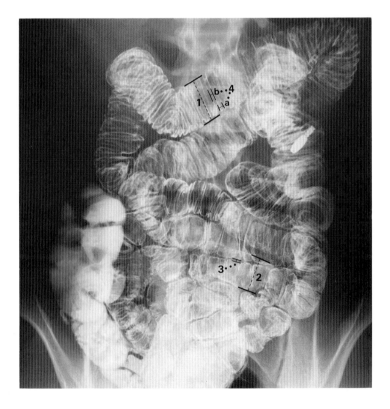

Checklist

Preliminary fluoroscopy	• No extraintestinal or intraperitoneal air
	• No air–fluid levels
	• No radiopaque foreign bodies
Technique	• Partial anesthesia of the nasopharynx
	• Tube is introduced perorally, aided by a guidewire
	• Tube is placed distal to the ligament of Treitz
	• 160 mL contrast medium and 1.5–2 L methylcellulose are instilled, until all intrapelvic small bowel loops and the terminal ileum are defined with adequate lucency
Shape	• Normal arrangement of small bowel loops with no fixed displacement
	• Unobstructed transit with normal distensibility of all segments
	• Normal luminal diameters (see below)
	• No circumscribed extraluminal or intraluminal constrictions or protrusions
	• Normal motility in all segments
	• Normal deformability of all palpable loops
Contours	• Smooth and sharp
	• Normal wall thickness (see below)
	• Normal fold thickness (see below)
	• Circular folds show a straight, parallel arrangement
	• No double contours or persistent niches
	• No spicules, no contrast pooling
	• Lumen and contours same as in rest of ileum
Ileocecal region	• Normal-appearing ileocecal valve with no excessive protrusion into the cecum

---

> **Important Data**
>
> 1. Jejunal diameter: ca. 3–4.5 cm (depending on filling pressure)
> 2. Ileal diameter: ca. 3 cm
> 3. Wall thickness: < 2 mm
> 4. Fold thickness: < 2 mm
>   The distance between the folds (a) is greater than the fold thickness (b)

Double-Contrast Examination of the Colon

The contrast enema should pass unobstructed through the rectum, sigmoid, and colon limbs, which display a normal shape and position.

All colon segments visualized in the double-contrast study show normal distensibility, normal haustrations, and normal luminal diameters. The films demonstrate a normal fine mucosal relief with smooth wall contours and a normal wall thickness.

The ileocecal region and appendix appear normal.

Interpretation

The colon appears normal, with no evidence of inflammatory changes or mass lesions.

Checklist

Preliminary fluoroscopy	• No extraintestinal or intraperitoneal air
	• No air–fluid levels
	• No radiopaque foreign bodies
	• No bowel contamination
Technique	• Contrast material is instilled into the colon per rectum (it is usually introduced to the hepatic flexure)
	• The colon is partially evacuated
	• Air is insufflated until all colon segments are expanded and the mucosa of the ascending colon is uniformly coated with contrast material
Shape	• Course (colon limbs)
	• No displacement of colic flexures, cecal pole, or sigmoid colon
	• No widening of the retrorectal space (see below)
	• Expansion of all colon segments
	• Normal luminal diameters (variable, compare colon segments with one another; no megacolon)
	• Normal haustrations
	• Motility
	– No rigid, widened, or constricted segments
	– No circumscribed impressions
	– No fistulous tracts

Mucosa	• Uniform, lucent mucosal coating en face
	• No persistent sites of contrast retention or filling defects (lymph follicles, granulations, ulcerations, tumors)
	• No fixed ring patterns (e.g., diverticulum, polyp)
	• No transverse or longitudinal striations, fine transverse lines, furrows (or innominate grooves)
Contours	• Smooth and sharp in tangential view
	• No wall irregularities (protrusions, spicules, double contours, niches, contrast pools, collar buttons)
	• Normal wall thickness
	• No wall constrictions
	• No stenosis
Cecum	• Mobility of cecal pole
	• Ileocecal valve:
	− Shape (intussusception?)
	− Thickness (inflammatory changes?)
	• Terminal ileum also visible?
Appendix	• Visualization, shape, position, length

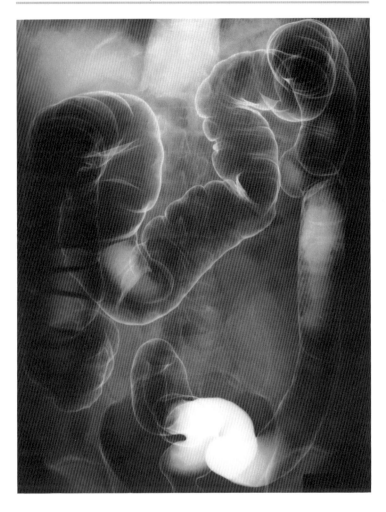

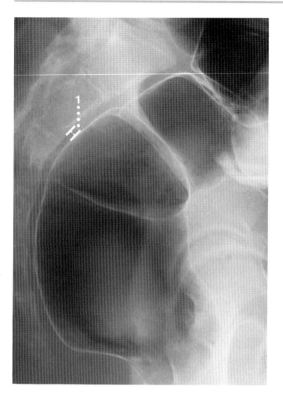

Important Data

1. Retrorectal space: usually less than 1 cm wide

Defecography

Contrast medium is introduced into the rectum and sigmoid through enema tubing, and then defecation is monitored fluoroscopically in the lateral projection.

The imaged wall contours appear smooth and normally distensible. The rectosigmoid junction and distal sigmoid present a normal shape, and the anorectal angle is normal prior to defecation. There is normal elevation of the rectum at the start of defecation. At this time the anorectal angle increases, and contrast medium flows from the rectum without obstruction. The subsequent film shows normal mucosal relief in the rectum.

Interpretation

The rectum and defecation process appear normal.

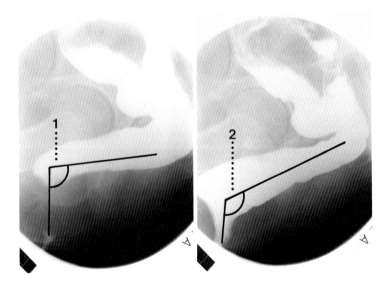

Checklist

Preliminary fluoroscopy	• No foreign bodies
	• No soft-tissue densities
	• No free intraperitoneal air
Technique	• Contrast medium is introduced into the rectum and sigmoid through an enema tube under fluoroscopic control
	• The tube is removed
	• Defecation is monitored fluoroscopically in the lateral projection
Shape, filling	• Rectosigmoid junction and distal sigmoid
	• Normal distensibility
	• Unobstructed passage of the contrast material
	• Normal luminal diameter
	• Smooth, sharp contours
	• No filling defects or constrictions
	• Sphincter is competent before and after tube removal
	• Anorectal angle (see below)
Defecation	• Increase in the anorectal angle
	• Adequate opening of the anal canal during defecation
	• Unobstructed evacuation of contrast material
	• No stenosis
	• No contrast pooling
	• No opacifying pouch-like recesses (e.g., rectocele)
	• Minimal contrast residues after evacuation
	• Normal mucosal relief after evacuation
	• Adequate sphincter closure after defecation

Important Data

Anorectal angle:
1. Sitting position at rest = 95–105°
2. During defecation = ca. 130–150°

Intravenous Contrast Studies

Intravenous Urography

Preliminary plain abdominal radiograph shows normal skeletal structures and soft-tissue shadows with no sign of abnormal calcifications.
After injection of the intravenous contrast medium, both kidneys show
homogeneous parenchymal opacification. There is normal timing of
contrast excretion, which is equal on both sides. The kidneys are normal
in shape, size, position, and axial orientation. Their outer contours are
smooth and clearly defined. The pyelocaliceal system appears normal.
The ureters are normal in shape, course, and caliber and permit unobstructed drainage of the contrast medium.
The bladder has a normal size and configuration, and its contours are
smooth.
There is no significant residual urine after micturition.

Interpretation

Both kidneys, the ureters, and the bladder appear normal at intravenous
urography.

Checklist

Plain radio-
graph
- Skeleton:
    - Shape (pelvis, lumbar spine, lower ribs)
    - Position (lumbar spine, pelvis)
- Psoas margins (smooth, sharp), position (symmetri-
cal)
- Inferior borders of the liver and spleen (smooth,
sharp, position)
- Bowel gas (distribution, contamination, air–fluid
levels)
- Kidneys: shape, position, size, delineation
- Soft tissues: calcifications, foreign bodies (projected
onto the kidneys, ureters, or bladder)

Technique	• Intravenous injection (infusion) of 1 mL (adults) to 3 mL (infants) of iodinated contrast medium per kg body weight (usually 60%)
Nephrogram	• Timing
	• Symmetry (equal on both sides)
	• Shape, size (see below)
	• Position (see below)
	• Renal orientation (parallel to psoas margins, see below)
	• Contours (smooth, sharp), no constriction, no circumscribed protrusion
	• Parenchymal structure (harmonious, no circumscribed lucency)
Excretion	• Pyelocaliceal system:
	− Time
	− Adequate, homogeneous opacification
	− Shape (calices: crescent-shaped, dendritic, ampullary, transitional type)
	− Calibers (finely tapered calices with no broadening, splaying, or thickening of the necks)
	− No reflux (pyelotubular)
	• Renal pelvis (single, ampullary? no circumscribed widening or narrowing, no filling defects)
	− Contours (smooth, sharp)
Ureters	• Course (see below), no abnormal displacement
	• Normal diameter (see below)
	• No circumscribed expansion due to obstruction (radiolucent stones, stenosis?)
	• Normal termination at the bladder
	• Unobstructed contrast drainage
	• Smooth, sharp contours
Bladder	• Concentric (round or oval)
	• No impressions or protrusions
	• Contours (smooth, sharp)
	• Homogeneous opacification with no filling defects or zones of increased density
	• No significant residual urine after voiding (see below)

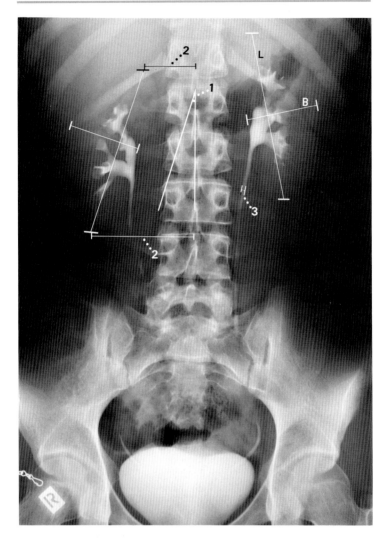

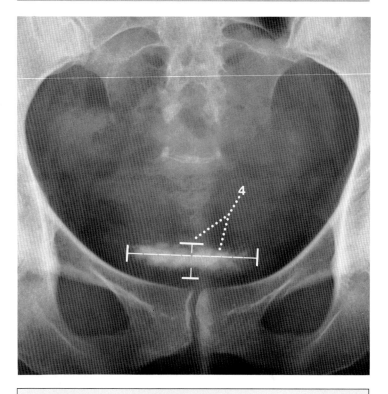

Important Data

Renal size: ca. 13 cm (length, L) × 6 cm (width, B)
Difference in lengths of right and left kidneys: ≤2 cm
Renal positions: left kidney ca. from T12 to L4; right kidney is up to 1 vertebral body lower than the left

1. *Inclination of renal axis:* ca. 10° (8–13°) relative to longitudinal body axis
2. *Distance of renal poles from central body axis:*
   (**a**) Upper pole ca. 4–5 cm
   (**b**) Lower pole ca. 6–9 cm

Course of ureter: along the spinal column, does not extend medially past the vertebral pedicles

3. *Ureteral diameter:* ca. 3–7 mm
4. *Residual urine:* elliptical bladder = ca. 5 cm × 3 cm (FFD 100)

Intravenous Cholecystocholangiography

The plain radiograph shows a normal hepatic shadow and a gallbladder devoid of calcific densities.

Film taken 30 minutes after contrast injection shows a normally positioned, uniformly opacified gallbladder of normal size with smooth wall contours. The intrahepatic bile ducts, cystic duct, and common bile duct show normal calibers, smooth margins, and adequate opacification with no filling defects.

Good contraction of the gallbladder is observed after a provocative meal.

Interpretation

Normal, positive cholecystocholangiogram.

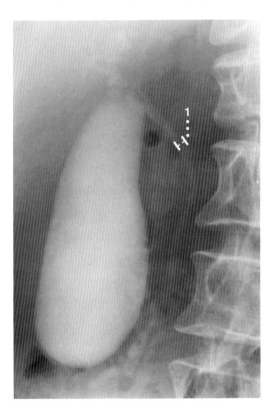

Checklist

Plain radiograph	• Normal hepatic shadow
	• Gallbladder (if visualized)
	• No calcifications or radiopaque foreign bodies
	• No air in the bile ducts
Technique	• Cholangiographic contrast medium (20 mL) is administered by short-term intravenous infusion (or injection)
	• Survey film or spot films for a clear projection (upright and recumbent; compression may be used after 30 min)
Gallbladder	• Shape (oblong ellipse, transverse)
	• Size (see below)
	• Position
	• Opacification
	• Homogeneous distribution of contrast medium
	• No filling defects
	• No densities
	• Contours (smooth, sharp)
	• No protrusions
Bile ducts	• Intrahepatic and extrahepatic
	• Delineation
	• Shape
	• Course
	• Luminal size (see below; no circumscribed narrowing or expansion)
	• Smooth wall contours
	• No filling defects or lucencies
Motility (gallbladder)	• Survey film or spot films, upright and recumbent, taken 30 (or 20) min after a provocative meal
	• Adequate, concentric contraction (usually by more than 1/3)
	• Homogeneous opacification, no filling defects
	• Smooth wall contours
	• Unobstructed drainage
	• No dilatation of bile ducts

Important Data

Gallbladder: size is variable (diameter greater than 5 cm)
1. *Common bile duct:* 3–9 mm in diameter
(up to 10 mm after cholecystectomy)

Endoscopic Retrograde Cholangiopancreaticography

Contrast medium is instilled into the pancreatic duct and common bile duct following peroral endoscopic catheterization of the papilla of Vater. Both ducts are normal in their position, length, and distribution, showing normal shape and contours to the level of the papilla. There is homogeneous opacification of all segments. Emptying of the pancreatic duct and common bile duct is not delayed.

The gallbladder shows normal opacification and no abnormalities.

Interpretation

Normal cholangiopancreaticogram.

Checklist

Technique
- The endoscope is introduced and advanced to the descending portion of the duodenum
- A catheter is passed into the papilla of Vater
- Contrast medium is injected

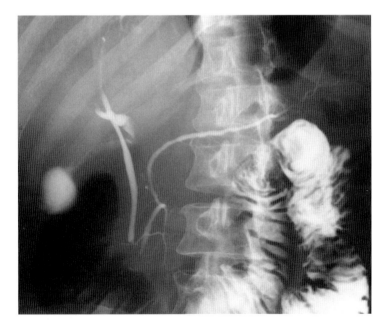

Pancreatic duct

Position	•	Normal, no displacement
Distribution	•	Normal "glandular" distribution, no absence of duct segments, no "string-of-beads" appearance (e.g., in pancreatitis)
Size	•	Tapers uniformly toward periphery (see below), no obstruction (e.g., by tumor, cyst, or inflammation), no stricture, no dilatation (e.g., prestenotic due to carcinoma), no segmental irregularities or local occlusion (e.g., acute recurring pancreatitis), no segmental ectasia
Duct shape	•	Contours: smooth, straight walls (not irregular or sacciform, not tortuous or dilated)
Density	•	Uniform, no calculi, no increased density (e.g., due to ectasia) or decreased density due to ductal narrowing
Function	•	No delay in emptying

Common bile duct

Course and position	•	Usually slightly convex to left, normal in number and anatomy
Size	•	Common bile duct tapers normally from its origin (both hepatic ducts and common bile duct are equal in size, see below), no circumscribed narrowing (stricture)
Duct shape	•	Contours: smooth, straight; no circumscribed change in diameter, especially near the papilla (e.g., prestenotic dilatation, discrete or segmental stenosis due to tumor or fibrosis)
Density	•	Uniform, no calculi, no increased density (e.g., due to ectasia) or decreased density due to ductal narrowing, lithiasis, or carcinoma
Function	•	Maximum density at 45 min, no delay in emptying
Gallbladder	•	Position, number, shape (septation), size, contours (smooth, diverticulum?), homogeneous opacification (no filling defect: sludge, stone, papilloma, carcinoma)

Important Data

Cystic duct: ca. 4 cm long
Common bile duct: normal diameter up to 10 mm

Arthrography

Arthrography of the Wrist

Preliminary plain radiograph shows normal shape and position of the imaged bones with a smooth, sharply defined radiocarpal joint space of normal width. There are no intra-articular or periarticular calcifications.

Under local anesthesia, 4 mL of iodinated contrast medium is injected percutaneously into the radiocarpal joint from the dorsal side.

Once the contrast medium is uniformly distributed, the radiocarpal joint appears normal in all respects. The proximal carpal bones and their ligaments form a smooth, sharply contoured articular surface on the distal side that is congruent with the cartilaginous surface of the radius and the normally shaped articular disk on the proximal side. Several intra-articular recesses are opacified with contrast medium at typical sites. There is no extravasation of contrast material into the intercarpal joints or soft tissues.

Interpretation

The wrist has a normal arthrographic appearance.

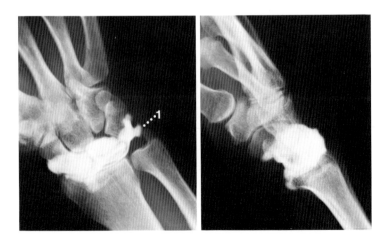

Checklist

Bones	• Distal radius, ulna, carpal bones:
	— Shape, position, structure, contours
	— Width of joint space
	— No intra-articular or periarticular calcifications
	• Soft-tissue envelope
Technique	• Under local anesthesia and fluoroscopic guidance, a needle is inserted into the joint space between the radius and scaphoid bone, usually from the dorsal side
	• 1.5–4 mL of iodinated contrast medium (usually 60%) is injected into the joint space
	• The contrast is uniformly distributed by active and passive wrist movements
	• Survey or spot films are obtained
Joint space	• Radiocarpal joint:
	— Shape
	— Width
	— Margins (smooth, sharp, intact)
	— No filling defects caused by intra-articular loose bodies
	— Distal articular surface: proximal carpal bones and ligaments
	– Proximal articular surface: radius and articular disk
	– Recesses (ulnar, proximal: prestyloid recess; radial, palmar: radial recess)
Neighboring joints	• Carpometacarpal joints
	• Intercarpal joints
	• Pisiform joint
	• Radioulnar joint (sacciform recess)
Cartilage	• Shape
	• Smooth, sharp contours with no discontinuities
	• No filling defect or niche

Important Data

1. Prestyloid recess

Arthrography of the Shoulder

The plain radiograph demonstrates normal-appearing skeletal structures. No intra-articular or periarticular calcifications are found.

Following local anesthesia, 10 mL of iodinated contrast medium is injected into the shoulder joint space from the anterior side. When the contrast medium is uniformly distributed, standard radiographs are obtained.

The shoulder joint space is normal in shape, size, and position. There is normal opacification of the normal-sized axillary recess and subscapular bursa. Other bursae are not visualized. The absence of contrast extravasation confirms the integrity of the rotator cuff. The capsule wall shows normal contours.

The tendon sheath of the long head of the biceps has a typical appearance. The articular cartilage on the joint surfaces is of normal thickness and has a normal shape and sharp margins.

Interpretation

The shoulder has a normal arthrographic appearance.

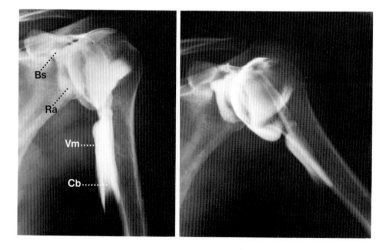

Checklist

Bones	• Shape, position (humeral head centered in glenoid)
	• Structure, contours (smooth, sharp)
	• Joint space (width, shape)
	• No intra-articular or periarticular calcifications
	• Soft-tissue envelope (intact, no swelling)
Technique	• Flat supine position
	• The shoulder is slightly abducted and externally rotated
	• The needle is inserted at a perpendicular angle at the approximate center of the joint space from the anterior side under fluoroscopic guidance (approx. 1 cm distal and lateral to the coracoid process)
	• 10–15 mL of iodinated contrast medium (e.g., 60%) is injected into the joint space
	• The contrast is uniformly distributed by active and passive joint movements
	• Standard radiographic views (AP with arm adducted and elevated, each view in internal and external rotation; bicipital groove)
Joint space	• Shape
	• Width (shoulder joint space)
	• Smooth margins
	• Intact rotator cuff:
	— Superior joint space: no craterlike niches, especially in the external rotation view
	— No contrast medium in the subacromial or subdeltoid bursa
	• No filling defects due to intra-articular loose bodies
Recesses	• *Axillary recess* (Ra)
	• *Subscapular bursa* (Bs) and subcoracoid recess (other recesses generally are not visualized)
	— Smooth walls of capsule and recesses
	— No contrast-filled niche
	— No irregularly shaped filling defect
	• *Intertubercular tendon sheath* (Vm):
	— Smooth margins
	• *Long biceps tendon sheath* (Cb):
	— Sharply defined, bandlike lucent line with smooth margins
	— No contrast extravasation into other recesses, soft tissues, or intermuscular intervals
Cartilage	• Shape, contours smooth and sharp
	• No filling defects or erosive lesions

Arthrography of the Knee

The knee joint and its bony structures show no abnormalities on the preliminary plain radiograph. There are no intra-articular or periarticular calcifications.

Following local anesthesia, 5 mL of iodinated contrast medium and 60 mL of air are injected into the superior recess of the knee joint from the lateral side. When the articular surfaces are uniformly coated with contrast material and the air is evenly distributed, spot films of the menisci are obtained.

All tangentially imaged portions of the medial and lateral menisci display a typical shape and have smooth, sharp margins. There are no abnormal contour defects or zones of contrast imbibition. There is no evidence of dislocation. The joint space and cartilage are of normal width and thickness, and their margins are smooth. The joint capsule is intact, has normal contours, and shows no signs of collateral ligament lesions. The bursae that communicate with the knee joint appear normal, and the cruciate ligaments appear as intact, linear filling defects within the opacified joint space.

Interpretation

The joint space, menisci, capsule, and ligaments of the knee joint appear normal.

Checklist

Bones	• Shape, position (varus, valgus)
	• Bone structure
	• Contours (smooth, sharp)
	• Joint space
	• No intra-articular or periarticular calcifications
	• Soft tissues
Technique	• The patella is elevated and pushed laterally
	• Under local anesthesia, the needle is inserted into the superior recess of the knee joint at the inferior patellar margin from the lateral side, level with the center of the patella
	• 5–10 mL of iodinated contrast medium (usually 60%) and 30–70 mL of air are injected
	• The contrast medium and air are uniformly distributed by active and passive knee movements

	• The knee is braced in position
	• Spot films are obtained (with the joint space spread open to get a clear projection of the menisci)
	• If necessary, a survey view or Frik view is obtained
Menisci	• Shape
	• Size (no deformity)
	• Position (no medial or lateral displacement)
	• Smooth, sharp borders
	• No circumscribed contour defect
	• No linear zones of opacification
Joint space	• Shape
	• Width (superior, inferior joint space)
	• No intra-articular loose body (opacified or causing a filling defect)
Cartilage	• Shape
	• Thickness (see below)
	• Smooth, sharp contours of femoral and tibial articular surfaces
	• No contour defects or erosions
Capsule	• Smooth, sharp borders
	• Collateral ligaments intact (medial ligament is fused with capsule and medial meniscus, lateral ligament is separate from capsule)
Bursae	• Suprapatellar, popliteal, semimembranous, gastrocnemus bursae (communicate with knee joint space)
	• Position
	• Smooth, sharp inner contours
Cruciate ligaments	• Linear filling defects (ca. 5–8 mm wide)
	• Shape
	• Position
	• Smooth, sharp contours
	• No contour defects (Tunnel view)

Medial meniscus   Lateral meniscus

	Medial meniscus	Lateral meniscus
Anterior horn (V)	Fused with the capsule on all sides Width: ca. 6 mm	Width: ca. 10 mm
Intermediate part (I)	Narrow meniscus, broad superior capsular recess	Broad meniscus, broad superior capsular recess
Posterior horn (P)	Broad meniscus (ca. 14 mm), narrow superior capsular recess	Not fused with capsule: slitlike lucent line, popliteus tendon

Important Data

1. Thickness of femoral cartilage: uniform 2–4 mm
2. Thickness of tibial cartilage: 1–2 mm on lateral plateau, 4–5 mm on medial plateau

Arthrography of the Ankle Joint

Imaged skeletal structures appear normal on the plain radiograph. The joint space is of normal width and has smooth, sharp borders. There are no intra-articular or periarticular calcifications.

Following local anesthesia, ca. 4 mL of iodinated contrast medium is injected into the ankle joint space from the anterior side. When the contrast has been uniformly distributed, standard radiographic views are obtained.

The ankle joint space displays a normal width and shape. Imaged portions of the articular cartilage have smooth, sharp margins. The opacified joint space shows a normal extent within the range of variation. The joint capsule and its recesses are intact and have smooth margins. There is no contrast extravasation into the soft tissues.

Interpretation

The ankle joint has a normal arthrographic appearance.

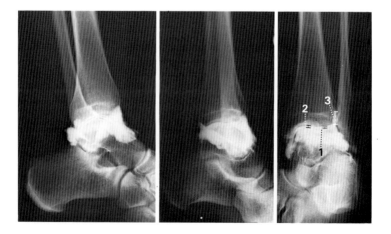

Checklist

Bones	• Shape
	• Position (ankle mortise, talus, joint angle)
	• Contours (smooth, sharp)
	• Width of joint space
	• No intra-articular or periarticular calcifications
	• Soft-tissue envelope (intact, no swelling)
Technique	• Under local anesthesia, the needle is inserted into the medial part of the joint space from the anterior side (fluoroscopic guidance may be used)
	• The needle is positioned medial to the tibialis anterior tendon with the ankle in slight internal rotation (avoid puncturing the dorsal pedal artery!)
	• 4–5 mL of iodinated contrast medium (usually 60%) is injected into the joint space
	• The contrast is uniformly distributed by active and passive ankle movements
	• Radiographs are taken immediately (because of absorption): AP and lateral views in internal and external rotation
Joint space	• Talocrural joint (inverted U shape)
	• Cartilage (smooth surfaces, normal thickness, see below; no filling defects or niches)
	• No intra-articular loose bodies
Capsule	• Smooth capsule wall (especially on lateral side: anterior and posterior talofibular ligaments and calcaneofibular ligament; on medial: deltoid ligament)
	• Smooth walls of anterior and posterior recesses (lateral view, normal size, see below)
	• Variant (in 5–15% of cases): posterior subtalar joint space
	• Connection with tendon sheaths (flexor hallucis and digitorum longus) is generally found on the medial side only

---

Important Data

1. Width of joint space = 1 mm
2. Thickness of articular cartilage = 2 mm
3. Syndesmotic recess (between distal tibia and fibula) = smaller than 2.5 cm

Arteriography

Internal Carotid Arteriography

Under local anesthesia, a 5-French selective catheter is introduced via the femoral artery using the Seldinger technique. After the carotid bifurcation is evaluated, the catheter tip is advanced into the internal carotid artery. Then serial arteriograms are obtained using DSA technique.

The films should show normal opacification of the internal carotid artery, which has smooth wall contours and a normal luminal diameter in its intra-cranial and extracranial segments. It divides normally into the anterior and middle cerebral arteries and their terminal branches, which are normal in their course and calibers.

A normal vascular pattern is seen during the capillary and venous phases, with good opacification of the internal cerebral veins, which appear centered in the sagittal projection. There is also unobstructed drainage of the contrast medium through the large cranial sinuses.

The course of the examination is uneventful.

Interpretation

The carotid artery has a normal angiographic appearance with no evidence of an intracranial mass lesion, peripheral vascular occlusions, or vascular malformations.

Checklist

Technique (e. g.)
- A 5-French catheter is introduced percutaneously via the femoral artery under local anesthesia
- The common carotid artery and carotid bifurcation are evaluated for plaques and stenoses
- The catheter tip is placed in the proximal part of the (right or left) internal carotid artery
- 4 mL of iodinated contrast medium is injected manually using DSA technique (nonionic contrast medium [concentration 150 mg iodine/mL] diluted 1:1 with 0.9% NaCl). (Caution: dilution with distilled water can cause osmotic hypotension.)

Vascular course and caliber	(described from central to peripheral):
Arterial phase	• *Internal carotid artery* (ci), carotid siphon:

- *Internal carotid artery* (ci), carotid siphon:
  - Ophthalmic artery (o)
  - Posterior communicating artery (co, if present)
- Anterior cerebral artery:
  - A1 segment not elevated (pituitary enlargement)
  - A2 segment not stretched (hydrocephalus)
  - No displacement (herniation)
  - "Handlebar mustache" (callosomarginal artery S— should be horizontal and bilaterally symmetrical)
  - Contralateral opacification via the anterior communicating artery
  - Pericallosal artery (p)
- *Middle cerebral artery:*
  - M1/M2 segment not displaced (elevated)
  - Lenticulostriate arteries, opercular part (M3 segment, no splaying of candelabra shape)
  - Loops of middle cerebral artery (see below)
  - Timely, homogeneous opacification
  - Course of vessels (no displacement)
  - Calibers (no circumscribed caliber change)
  - Smooth, sharp wall contours
  - No vascular cutoff, no pathological vessels
  - No premature venous drainage (e.g., tumors and A-V fistulae)

Venous phase

- Timely opacification of superior sagittal sinus (Sss) with thalamostriate veins (Vt), internal cerebral vein (Vci), great cerebral vein (Vcm), straight sinus (Sr), sinus confluence (Cs), transverse sinus (St), and sigmoid sinus (Ss):
  - Timely, uniform opacification (no filling defect)
  - Course: no displacement of internal cerebral veins
  - Caliber: no stenosis
  - Unobstructed contrast drainage

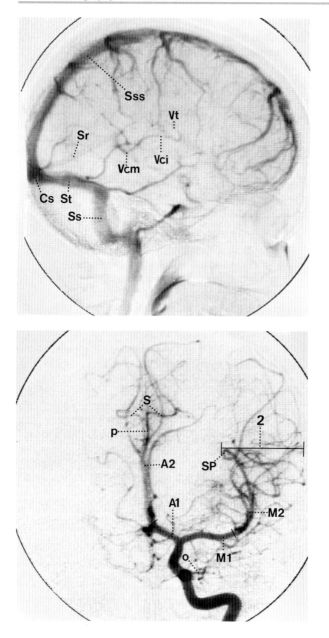

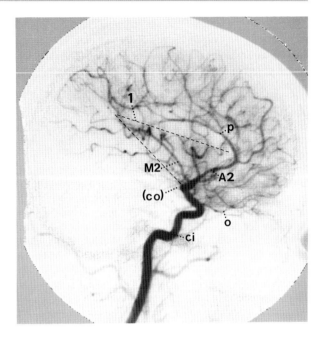

Important Data

1. Insular loops of middle cerebral artery on one line (sylvian triangle)
2. Distance from sylvian point (insular region, SP) to inner table of skull = ca. 30–40 mm

Vertebral Arteriography

Under local anesthesia, a 5-French catheter is introduced via the femoral artery using the Seldinger technique. The catheter tip is placed in the vertebral artery, and serial films are obtained using DSA technique.

The films should demonstrate a normal course of the upper cervical part of the vertebral artery, retrograde opacification of the contralateral vertebral artery, and opacification of both posterior inferior cerebellar arteries. The tonsillar loops are not displaced from the foramen magnum. The choroidal point is normally positioned.

The branches to the cerebellar vermis run on the midline. The basilar artery runs on the midline and is not pressed against the clivus. Both superior cerebellar arteries and posterior cerebral arteries pursue a normal course around the brain stem. The branches of the superior cerebellar artery are not splayed. The perforating thalamic arteries and posterior choroidal arteries are unremarkable. During the venous phase, the paramedian hemispheric arteries are visualized with no sign of displacement. The precentral vein of the cerebellum terminates normally in the great cerebral vein.

The course of the examination is uneventful.

Interpretation

The vertebral artery and the basilar artery and its branches have a normal angiographic appearance. In particular, there is no evidence of an intracranial mass lesion, peripheral vascular occlusions, or vascular malformations.

Checklist

Technique
(e. g.)

- A 5-French catheter is introduced percutaneously via the femoral artery under local anesthesia
- The origin of the vertebral artery is evaluated for plaques and stenosis (site of predilection!)
- The catheter tip is placed in the proximal part of the (right or left) vertebral artery (or in the subclavian artery near the origin of the vertebral artery)
- e. g. 3 mL of iodinated contrast medium is injected manually using DSA technique (nonionic contrast medium [concentration 150 mg iodine/mL] diluted 1:1 with 0.9% NaCl) (Caution: Dilution with distilled water can cause osmotic hypotension)

Vascular course
and caliber (described from central to peripheral):

Arterial
phase
- Cervical segment of the vertebral artery
- Intracranial segment of the vertebral artery (stenosis, plaques? site of predilection!)
- Posterior inferior cerebellar artery (PICA, Pi)
- Tonsillar loops not displaced from foramen magnum
- Basilar artery (B, not pressed against clivus, not displaced posteriorly, see below)
- Anterior inferior cerebellar artery (AICA, Ai)
- Superior cerebellar artery (branches not splayed, Cs)
- Perforating thalamic arteries (T)
- Posterior cerebral artery (Cp)
- Posterior communicating artery (if present, Co)
- Occipitotemporal artery (Ot)
- Internal occipital (calcarine) artery (Oi)
- Parieto-occipital artery (Po)
- Choroidal point (see below)
- Timely, homogeneous opacification (thrombosis? Caution: layering effect)
- Course of vessels (no displacement)
- Calibers (no circumscribed caliber change)
- Smooth, sharp wall contours
- No vascular cutoff, no pathological vessels
- No premature venous drainage (e.g., tumors and A-V fistulae)

Venous
phase
- Prepontine veins (Vpp)
- Precentral vein (Vp)
- Great cerebral vein (Vcm)
- Straight sinus (Sr)
- Sinus confluence (Cs)
- Inferior cerebellar veins (vermian and hemispheric veins, Vci)
- Transverse sinus (St)
- Sigmoid sinus (Ss):
- Timely, uniform opacification (no filling defect)
- Course: no displacement of vessels
- Caliber: no stenosis
- Unobstructed contrast drainage

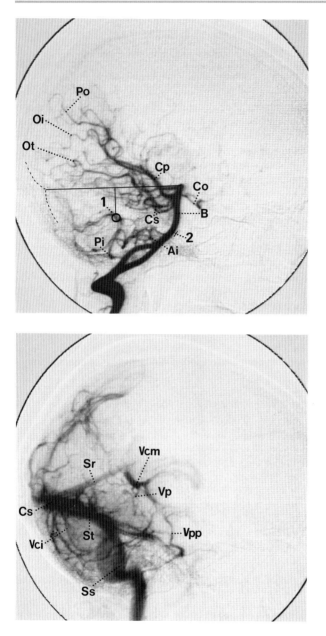

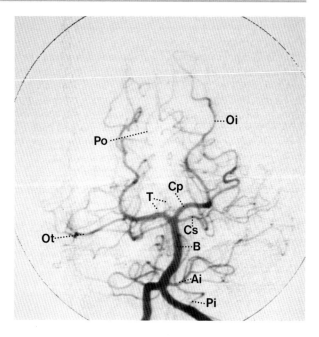

Important Data

1. *Choroidal point:* located on the perpendicular that bisects a line connecting the tip of the basilar artery with the internal occipital protuberance
2. Distance from basilar artery to clivus = > 1 mm

Arch Aortography

A pigtail catheter is introduced via the femoral artery under local anesthesia (Seldinger technique) and is advanced into the proximal ascending aorta. Iodinated contrast medium (60 mL) is injected under pressure at a flow rate of 25 mL/s, and serial films are obtained.

The aortic arch displays smooth walls and a normal configuration. Its lumen is of normal caliber and homogeneously opacified. The supraaortic vessels and their branches display a normal course and arrangement, smooth wall contours, and no intraluminal filling defects.

The venous phase of the arteriogram is normal.

The course of the examination is uneventful.

Interpretation

The aortic arch and the vessels arising from it have a normal angiographic appearance.

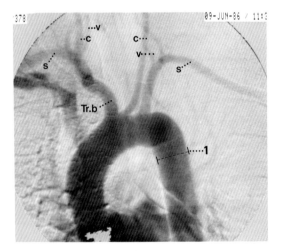

Important Data

1. Caliber of aorta = ca. 2–4 cm

Checklist

Technique (e. g.)	• A 5-French pigtail catheter is introduced via the femoral artery over a guidewire under local anesthesia (Seldinger technique)
	• The catheter tip is placed in the ascending aorta between the origin of the aorta and the brachiocephalic trunk (ca. 4 cm distal to the valve)
	• 60 mL of iodinated contrast medium (usually nonionic) is injected under pressure at a flow rate of 25–30 mL/s
	• Serial films are obtained (with left side elevated)
Plain radiograph	• Normal thoracic anatomy (vascular shadows, mediastinum, lung, skeleton)
	• No abnormal calcifications or radiopaque foreign bodies
Vessels	(described from central to peripheral)
Arterial phase	• *Ascending aorta* (aortic valve?), aortic arch, descending aorta:
	— Course
	— Caliber (see below), no narrowing or dilatation
	— Vessel wall (smooth), no double contours
	— No niches or impressions
	— No contrast extravasation
	• *Main branches:*
	— Right: brachiocephalic trunk (Tr.b) with division into subclavian (s) and carotid arteries (c), vertebral artery (v)
	— Left: carotid artery (c), subclavian artery (s), vertebral artery (v) (and perhaps the internal mammary artery):
	— Course (no displacement)
	— Calibers (side-to-side comparison), no abrupt caliber changes, no stenosis
	— No filling defects, no ulcerations
	— Contours (smooth, sharp)
	— No pathologic vessels or vascular cutoffs
	— No atypical vascular origins
Venous phase	• Unobstructed contrast drainage
	• No contrast retention
	• No flow reversal or steal effect
Course of examination	• Well tolerated by the patient
	• Good pedal pulses, no complications (dissection, hematoma, palsy, etc.)

Pulmonary Arteriography

A total of 60 mL of a nonionic contrast medium is mechanically injected via a cubital vein, and serial films are obtained using DSA technique.

The pulmonary trunk has a normal appearance and shows a normal bifurcation. The upper, middle, and lower lobar vessels in both lungs are complete, have normal calibers, smooth walls, and a normal course. A homogeneous pattern is seen in the capillary phase. Contrast drainage is not premature or obstructed.

The veins appear normal in their course, calibers, and wall contours.

Interpretation

The pulmonary vessels have a normal angiographic appearance, with no evidence of a circumscribed perfusion deficit.

Checklist

Technique (e. g.)	• Cubital vein puncture may be used (for DSA), or a 5-Fr pigtail catheter may be passed via the femoral vein into the proximal inferior vena cava using Seldinger technique
	• 60 mL of iodinated contrast medium (usually nonionic) is mechanically injected under pressure at a flow rate of 25 mL/s
	• Serial films are obtained
Plain radiograph	• Normal thoracic anatomy (vascular shadows, mediastinum, lung, skeleton)
	• No abnormal calcifications or foreign bodies

Vascular course
and caliber (described from central to peripheral):

Arterial phase
- Pulmonary trunk
  - *Left pulmonary artery* (segmental branches A1–A10):
    - Upper lobe: 4–8 arteries = A1–A5
    - Lower lobe: interlobar part = A6, basal part:
      (a) Mediobasal group (= A7+A8)
      (b) Laterobasal group (=A9+A10)
  - *Right pulmonary artery* (segmental branches A1–A10):
    - Upper lobe: superior trunk, 1–3 upper lobe arteries, usually 3: apical, posterior, anterior branches = A1–A3
    - Middle lobe: either 1 or 2 branches A4+A5 (each in about 50% of cases)
    - Lower lobe: inferior apical lobar branch = A6 Basal part: division into A7–A10
- Course (no displacement)
- Caliber (side-to-side comparison)
- No abrupt caliber changes or stenosis
- No filling defects, no ulcerations
- Contours (smooth, sharp)
- No pathological vessels or vascular cutoffs
- No atypical vascular origins

Capillary phase
- Homogeneous perfusion pattern
- No circumscribed perfusion deficits

Venous phase
- Normal timing
- Normal cardiac chambers (left atrium = LA)
- Unobstructed contrast drainage
- No contrast retention or lacunae

Course of examination
- Well tolerated by the patient
- Good pedal pulses, no complications (dissection, hematoma, palsy, etc.)

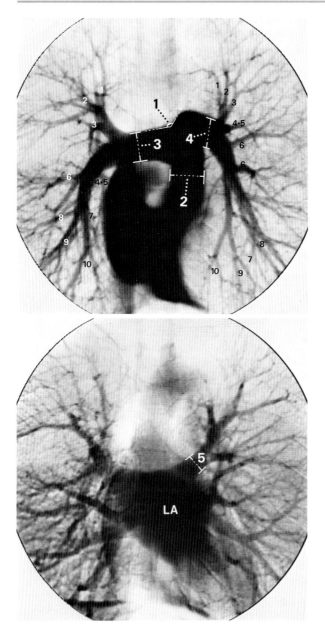

Important Data

1. *Bifurcation angle* of pulmonary trunk = 130–150° (superiorly open angle)

Vascular calibers:

2. Pulmonary trunk = 2.2–3.5 cm
3. Right pulmonary artery = 2–2.3 cm
4. Left pulmonary artery = 1.8–2.1 cm
5. Pulmonary veins = 1.4–1.6 cm

Celiac Trunk Arteriography

The celiac trunk is selectively catheterized via the femoral artery under local anesthesia using the Seldinger technique, then 50 mL of iodinated contrast medium is mechanically pressure-injected at a flow rate of 10 mL/s.

The preliminary plain radiograph shows no significant abnormalities.

The serial arteriograms show a typical, normal-caliber origin of the celiac trunk from the abdominal aorta. The trunk divides into the splenic artery, common hepatic artery, and left gastric artery, which are normally distributed and show normal, timely opacification. Their course, calibers, and wall contours are unremarkable.

The parenchymal phase is characterized by a homogeneous pattern of contrast distribution with normal visualization of the parenchymatous organs.

Venous opacification is distinct and not premature, and the drainage phase is normal.

The course of the examination is uneventful.

Interpretation

The celiac trunk and its branches have a normal angiographic appearance.

Checklist

Technique
- A selective catheter is introduced over a guidewire via the femoral artery under local anesthesia (Seldinger technique)
- The catheter tip is placed in the celiac trunk under fluoroscopic control, and a trial injection is performed
- 50 mL of iodinated contrast medium (usually non-ionic) is injected under pressure at a flow rate of 10 mL/s
- Serial radiographs or DSA images (20–30 mL contrast) are obtained

Plain radiograph	• Normal anatomy of the lumbar spine
	• No abnormal calcifications or foreign bodies
	• No soft-tissue masses

Vascular course and caliber

Arterial phase (described from central to peripheral):

- Celiac trunk (Tr.c): typical origin (see below)
  - *Splenic artery* (1): course (tortuous, branches at splenic hilum)
  - *Common hepatic artery* (hc):
    (a) Proper hepatic artery: left gastric artery (*), left hepatic artery (hs), right hepatic artery (hd)
    (b) Gastroduodenal artery (gd)
  - *Left gastric artery* (third vessel arising from celiac trunk, usually of large caliber [not shown in figure]):
    - Gastroepiploic artery (ge)
- Course (no displacement)
- No vascular cutoff
- No pathological vessels or contrast extravasation
- No abrupt caliber changes or stenosis
- Homogeneous opacification, smooth and sharp contours, no filling defects or ulcerations

Parenchymal phase
- Pattern of contrast distribution
- Normal organ size, contours, position (see below)

Venous phase
- Course of veins:
- Splenic vein (VI, straight course)
- Portal vein (Vp)
- No vascular displacement, no collaterals
- No premature venous opacification
- Calibers, inner contours (smooth, sharp)
- Unobstructed contrast drainage, no contrast retention

Course of examination
- No complications (e.g., contrast allergy, hematoma, hemorrhage, palsy, vascular injury)
- Good pedal pulses

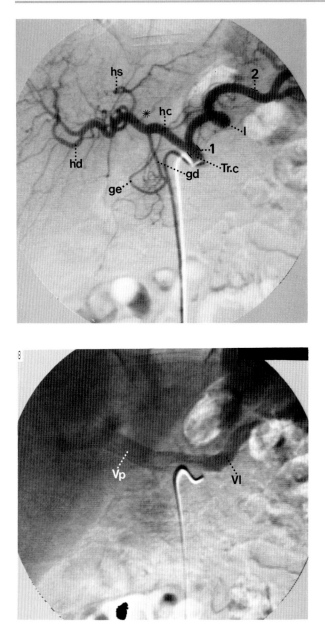

Important Data

Vascular calibers:
1. Celiac trunk = 5–10 mm
2. Splenic artery = 5–10 mm
Origin of celiac trunk: at level of T12
Dimensions of spleen: 7 cm (length) × 12 cm (width) (× magnification factor!)
Position of spleen: lower pole at level of L1–L3
Liver: between diaphragm leaflet and inferior costal margin; does not extend below level of kidney

Superior Mesenteric Arteriography

The superior mesenteric artery is selectively catheterized via the trans-femoral approach under local anesthesia using the Seldinger technique. Then 50 mL of iodinated contrast medium is mechanically pressure-injected at a flow rate of 10 mL/s, and serial films are obtained.

The preliminary plain radiograph shows no significant abnormalities.

The arteriograms show a typical, normal-caliber origin of the superior mesenteric artery from the abdominal aorta at the L1 level. The vessel shows a normal branching pattern with normal, timely opacification of the vessels supplying the small and large intestine. The vessels have smooth wall contours and are normal in course and caliber. There are no signs of contrast extravasation or A-V fistulae.

The parenchymal phase is characterized by a normal, homogeneous pattern of contrast distribution.

The veins are clearly opacified during the venous phase, appearing normal in their course, calibers, and contours. There is no obstruction of contrast drainage into the superior mesenteric vein and portal vein.

The course of the examination is uneventful.

Interpretation

The superior mesenteric artery and its branches have a normal angiographic appearance during the arterial, capillary, and venous phases of the study.

Checklist

Technique (e. g.)	• A selective catheter is introduced over a guidewire via the femoral artery under local anesthesia (Seldinger technique)
	• The catheter tip is placed in the superior mesenteric artery
	• 50 mL of iodinated contrast medium is injected under pressure at a flow rate of 10 mL/s
	• Serial radiographs (15 × 1 films/s) or DSA images (20–30 mL contrast) are obtained
Plain radiograph	• Normal anatomy of the lumbar spine
	• No abnormal calcifications or radiopaque foreign bodies
	• No soft-tissue masses

Vascular course and caliber	(described from central to peripheral):

Arterial phase	• Superior mesenteric artery (ms):
	  — Typical origin (see below)
	  — Course (descends in a slight S-shaped curve)
	  — Caliber (see below), no constrictions, dilatations, or filling defects
	  — Vessel walls (smooth, sharp)
	• Branching pattern of vessels to small and large intestine:
	  — Superior mesenteric artery (ms)
	  — Right gastroepiploic artery (if visualized)
	  — Jejunal arteries (j)
	  — Ileocolic artery (ic)
	  — Ileal arteries (i)
	  — Middle colic artery (cm) and right colic artery (cd)
	• Intramural distribution pattern
	• Course: no displacements
	• No vascular cutoff, pathological vessels, or contrast extravasation
	• No abrupt caliber changes or stenosis
	• No filling defects or ulcerations
	• Contours (smooth, sharp)
	• No A-V fistulae

Parenchymal phase Venous phase	• Uniform staining of bowel walls • No circumscribed areas of increased blood flow • Normal timing of venous opacification • Course of veins (parallel to arteries) • Normal opacification of right colic vein (Vcd), jejunal veins (Vvj), ilial veins (Vvi), superior mesenteric vein (Vms), and portal vein (Vp) • Calibers (larger than arteries) • Smooth, sharp contours • Unobstructed contrast drainage, no contrast retention
Course of examination	• No complications (e.g., contrast allergy, hemorrhage, neurovascular injury)

Important Data

1. Caliber of superior mesenteric artery = ca. 4–6 mm
   Origin of superior mesenteric artery: at L1 level

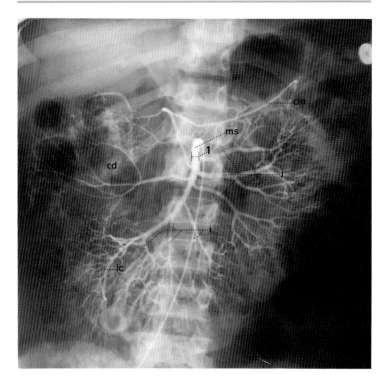

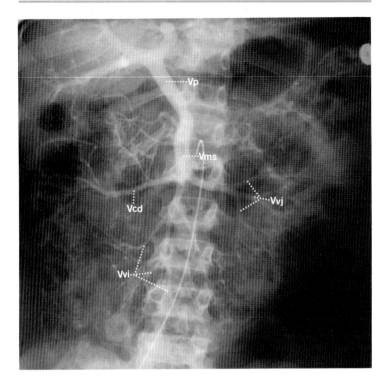

Renal Arteriography

A 5-French pigtail catheter is introduced via the femoral artery into the abdominal aorta under local anesthesia using the Seldinger technique. The catheter tip is advanced to the T12/L1 level, and serial films are obtained while 40 mL of nonionic contrast medium is mechanically pressure-injected at a flow rate of 22 mL/s.

The plain abdominal radiograph shows no significant abnormalities.

The arteriograms show a normal course and caliber of the abdominal aorta. The origins of the unpaired visceral arteries, if visualized, are normal.

The renal arterial trunks arise at the level of the first lumbar vertebral body and divide normally into the individual segmental arteries. The course, caliber, and wall contours of these vessels are normal.

The capillary, venous, and parenchymal phases show normal timing on both sides and are unremarkable. Both kidneys are normal in their position, shape, size, and borders.

Interpretation

The renal arteriogram demonstrates a normal vascular system.

Checklist

Technique (e. g.)	• A 5-French pigtail catheter is introduced over a guidewire via the femoral artery under local anesthesia (Seldinger technique)
	• The catheter tip is placed in the aorta above the origin of the renal arteries under fluoroscopic control
	• 40–50 mL of iodinated contrast medium (usually nonionic) is injected under pressure at a flow rate of 22 mL/s
	• Serial films (3 × 2 and 4 × 1 films/s) are obtained
Plain radiograph	• Normal anatomy of the lumbar spine
	• No abnormal calcifications or radiopaque foreign bodies

Vascular course
and caliber (described from central to peripheral):

Arterial phase	● *Abdominal aorta:* (descends in an almost straight course to left of spinal column; bifurcation)
	— Caliber (see below)
	— No abrupt caliber changes, no stenosis, no wall irregularities
	● *Renal arteries:*
	— Number (paired), no accessory polar arteries
	— Origin (see below)
	— Branching pattern (anterior and posterior main branches, segmental and subsegmental arteries)
	— Caliber (see below)
	— No abrupt caliber changes, no stenosis, no wall irregularities
	— No pathological vessels, lacunae, or vascular cutoffs
	— Course (no stretching or splaying of the vessels)
Parenchymal phase	● Normal timing (equal on both sides, see below)
	● Homogeneous opacification of the renal cortex
	● Thickness of the renal cortex (see below)
	● Renal shape and size (see below)
	● Axial orientation (parallel to psoas muscle)
	● Contours (smooth, sharp)
	● No circumscribed notching or protrusion
Venous phase	● Normal timing (see below), equal on both sides
	● Normal course of veins (parallel to arteries)
	● Calibers (thicker than arteries), equal on both sides
	● No filling defects
Late venous phase	● No lacunae
	● No circumscribed contrast retention
	● Unobstructed contrast drainage
Course of examination	● Well tolerated by the patient
	● Good pedal pulses

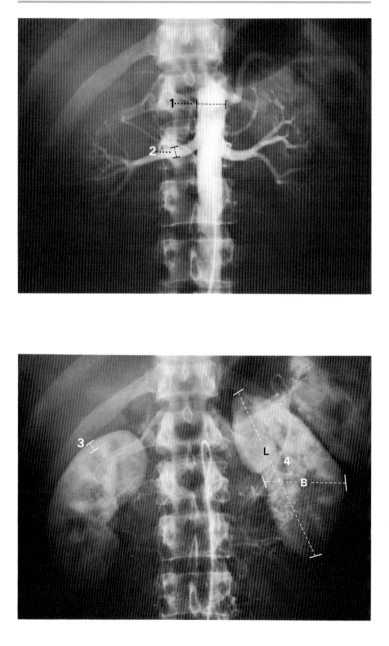

Important Data

Vascular calibers:
1. Abdominal aorta: ca. 2–4 cm
2. Renal artery: 4.5–10 mm
3. *Cortical thickness:* ca. 4–5 mm
4. *Renal dimensions:* ca. 12–16 cm (length, L) × 6 cm (width, W)
   Difference in lengths: ≤ 2 cm
   Origin of renal arteries: ca. the L1–L2 level
   Parenchymal phase: onset at ca. 2 seconds postinjection
   Venous phase: onset at ca. 3–5 seconds postinjection

Peripheral Arteriography of the Lower Extremity

A 5-French pigtail catheter is passed via the femoral artery into the distal abdominal aorta under local anesthesia using Seldinger technique. Serial films are obtained with table incrementation while 80 mL of non-ionic contrast medium is mechanically pressure-injected at a flow rate of 11 mL/s.

The plain abdominal radiograph shows no significant abnormalities.

The serial films demonstrate a normal course and caliber of the abdominal aorta, the aortic bifurcation, and the common, internal, and external iliac arteries.

Both common femoral arteries have normal calibers and smooth walls and divide normally into three femoral arteries. The deep and circumflex femoral arteries are of normal caliber.

There is normal visualization of the superficial femoral arteries, which are continuous distally with the popliteal arteries. The three lower leg arteries arise normally, have normal calibers and smooth walls, and can be traced distally to the level of the malleoli and the dorsum of the foot.

Interpretation

The arterial system of the lower extremity appears normal.

Checklist

Technique (e. g.)	• A 5-French pigtail catheter is introduced over a guidewire via the femoral artery under local anesthesia (Seldinger technique)
	• The catheter tip is placed in the distal abdominal aorta above the bifurcation
	• 80 mL of iodinated contrast medium is mechanically injected under pressure at a flow rate of 11 mL/s
	• Serial films are obtained with 4 table incrementations (= 5 filming stations, each with 2 × 1 film/s)
Plain radiograph	• Normal anatomy of the lumbar spine
	• No abnormal calcifications or radiopaque foreign bodies

Vascular course and caliber	(described from central to peripheral):

Arterial phase	● *Abdominal aorta:*
	 (descends in an almost straight course to left of spinal column; bifurcation, see below)
	   — Caliber (see below)
	   — No abrupt caliber changes, no stenosis
	   — Smooth wall contours with no filling defects
	 ● Common iliac artery (ic)
	 ● External iliac artery (ie)
	 ● Internal iliac artery (ii)
	 ● Superior gluteal artery (gs)
	 ● Common femoral artery (fco)
	 ● Superficial femoral artery (fs)
	 ● Circumflex femoral artery (fci)
	 ● Deep femoral artery (fp)
	 ● Popliteal artery (p)
	 ● Anterior tibial artery (ta)
	 ● Posterior tibial artery (tp) (lateral on internal rotation view)
	 ● Peroneal artery (f)
	 ● Malleolar arteries
	 ● Dorsal pedal artery
	 ● Arcuate and medial plantar arteries (if visualized):
	   — Course
	   — Caliber (see below) (tapering, side-to-side comparison)
	   — No abrupt caliber changes or stenosis
	   — No filling defects or ulcerations
	   — Contours (smooth, sharp)
	   – No pathological vessels or vascular cutoffs

Venous phase	● Unobstructed contrast drainage ● No contrast retention, no lacunae
Course of examination	● No complications (contrast allergy, hemorrhage, neurovascular injury) ● Good pedal pulses

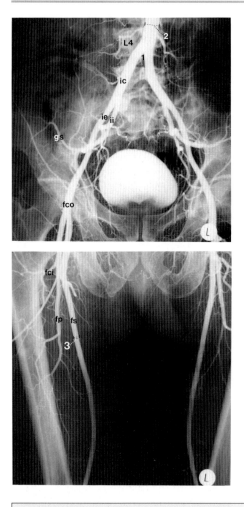

Important Data

1. *Bifurcation:* ca. at L4–L5 level
Vascular calibers:
2. Abdominal aorta = ca. 2–4 cm
3. Superficial femoral artery = 0.7–1.5 cm
4. Popliteal artery = 0.6–1 cm

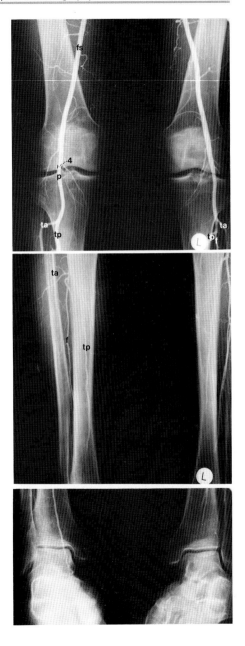

Venography

Inferior Cavography

A catheter is introduced via the right femoral vein into the inferior vena cava under local anesthesia and advanced to the level of the confluence. Serial films are obtained while 50 mL of iodinated contrast medium is injected under pressure at a flow rate of 15 mL/s.

The inferior vena cava is normally positioned and displays smooth wall contours and a normal luminal diameter throughout its length. Venous drainage is unobstructed, and there are no abnormal intraluminal filling defects.

Interpretation

The inferior vena cava appears normal.

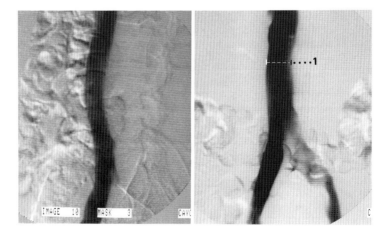

Checklist

Technique (e. g.)	• A straight catheter (or 5-French pigtail catheter) is introduced via the femoral vein into the inferior vena cava under local anesthesia and advanced to the level of the confluence
	• 50 mL of iodinated contrast medium is injected under pressure at a flow rate of 15 mL/s
	• Serial venograms (usually biplane) are obtained, or manual injection is performed using DSA technique
Plain radiograph	• Normal anatomy of the lumbar spine
	• No abnormal calcifications or radiopaque foreign bodies
Vascular course and caliber	• Ascends in an almost straight course to right of spinal column
	• Caliber (see below)
	• No luminal narrowing or dilatation
	• Homogeneous opacification (flow phenomenon!)
	• No filling defect (pseudothrombus artifact)
	• Contours smooth and sharp
	• Unobstructed contrast drainage
	• No collaterals
	• No intraluminal foreign bodies

Important Data

1. Caliber of inferior vena cava: 20–30 mm

Venography of the Upper Extremity

A nonionic contrast medium (40 mL) is injected through a superficial vein at the wrist, and spot films are obtained under fluoroscopic control.

The deep veins of the forearm show complete, homogeneous opacification with smooth wall contours and intact valves. There is unobstructed drainage into the brachial veins. A second injection demonstrates a normal superficial venous system. There is free drainage through the axillary, subclavian, and brachiocephalic veins and the superior vena cava. When adequately opacified, these vessels display normal calibers and smooth wall contours.

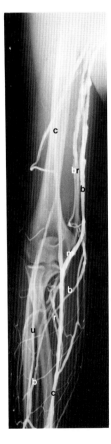

Interpretation

The imaged veins of the upper extremity appear normal.

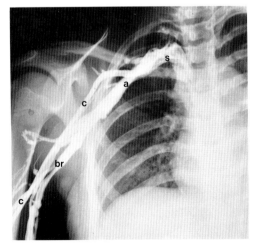

Checklist

Technique (e. g.)	• Superficial venipuncture at the wrist
	• 40–60 mL of a nonionic contrast medium is manually injected with and without the use of a tourniquet
	• A tourniquet is used for assessing the patency of the deep veins (e.g., thrombosis); it is not used for imaging the superficial veins (e.g., assessing venous status before creating a dialysis shunt)
	• Spot films are obtained under fluoroscopic control (forearm, upper arm, shoulder, upper chest)
Preliminary fluoroscopy	• Normal skeletal structures and soft tissues
	• No calcifications or radiopaque foreign bodies
Vascular course and caliber	• Normal visualization of the superficial and deep venous systems
	— Ulnar veins (u)
	— Radial veins (r)
	— Median antebrachial vein (m)
	— Basilic vein (b)
	— Cephalic vein (c)
	— Brachial veins (br)
	— Axillary vein (a)
	— Subclavian vein (s)
	— Superior vena cava
	• Superficial venous system (without a tourniquet):
	— Reticular, no vascular cutoff
	• Course (no displacement)
	• Caliber (no narrowing or dilatation, no filling defects)
	• Smooth wall contours
	• Competent valves
	• Unobstructed contrast drainage through the axillary, subclavian and brachiocephalic veins and superior vena cava (should not be completely opacified)
	• No cutoff of the contrast column, no contrast stasis
	• No collateral vessels (course, caliber)

Venography of the Lower Extremity

With a tourniquet on the ankle, a superficial dorsal pedal vein is punctured and 60 mL of iodinated contrast medium is manually injected. Spot films are then obtained under fluoroscopic control. The films show unobstructed contrast drainage through the smoothly marginated deep venous systems of the upper and lower leg, which have a competent valvular apparatus. Incompetent communicating veins are not demonstrated.

Films taken during a Valsalva maneuver demonstrate normal drainage from the saphenous trunks.

Films at the pelvic level also demonstrate normal venous anatomy with no evidence of filling defects.

Interpretation

The deep venous system of the lower extremity appears normal, with no evidence of valvular insufficiency.

Checklist

Technique	• With the patient in an inclined position and an ankle tourniquet in place, a superficial dorsal pedal vein (usually the dorsal vein of the big toe) is punctured
	• 40–60 mL of iodinated contrast medium (usually nonionic) is manually injected
	• Spot films are taken under fluoroscopic control in internal and external rotation (30°), and lateral views are taken of the knee and lower leg
	• A Valsalva maneuver is performed to test valvular competence (e.g., of the long saphenous vein)
Preliminary fluoroscopy	• Normal skeletal structures and soft tissues
	• No calcifications or radiopaque foreign bodies
Vascular course and caliber	• *Deep venous system:*
	— Anterior tibial veins (ta, usually double, lateral on internal rotation view)
	— Posterior tibial veins (tp, double, medial)
	— Peroneal vein (f, usually solitary, located between anterior and posterior tibial veins, aids in differentiating physiological venous ectasia)
	— Popliteal vein (p)

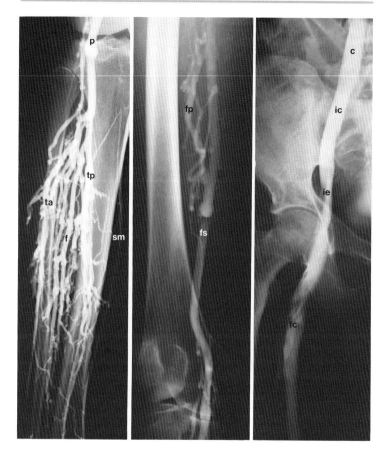

- Superficial femoral vein (fs)
- Profunda femoris vein (fp) (if visualized)
- Common femoral vein (fc)
- External iliac vein (ie)
- Common iliac vein (ic)
- Inferior vena cava (c)
- *Superficial venous system:*
  - Long saphenous vein (sm) (usually solitary, medial, telescope sign of competent valves before termination at femoral vein, no reflux during Valsalva maneuver)

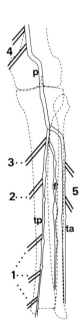

- Short saphenous vein (posterior in lower leg, opens into popliteal vein ca. 5–7 cm above knee joint)
- Gastrocnemius veins (usually 2–4, have more valves than the short saphenous vein)

- *Perforating veins:*
  - Medial side
    1. 3 Cockett veins (distal lower leg between posterior tibial vein and long saphenous vein or posterior arch vein)
    2. Sherman vein (between Cockett and Boyd veins)
    3. Boyd vein (below knee between posterior tibial vein and long saphenous vein)
    4. Dodd veins (3–5 pairs in lower third of thigh, between superficial femoral vein and long saphenous vein)
  - Lateral side
    5. Lateral perforating veins (between long saphenous vein and anterior tibial vein)
- *Muscle veins:*
  - Soleus and gastrocnemius veins
- Course (no displacement, tortuosity)
- Caliber (no narrowing, dilatation, ectasia, aneurysms)
- Wall contours (smooth)
- No filling defects
- Venous valves intact and competent
- Competent perforating veins (paired, spindle shape, valves intact, acute termination angle, course not horizontal!)
- No reflux into long saphenous vein during Valsalva maneuver
- Unobstructed contrast drainage (no cutoff of contrast column, no collateral circulation)
- No tortuosity of imaged superficial veins

Special Examinations

Thoracic Myelography

A high lumbar puncture is performed, and 10 mL of nonionic contrast medium is injected into the spinal subarachnoid space. Radiographs are then obtained under fluoroscopic control and are supplemented as needed by tomographic views. The preliminary plain radiograph of the lumbar spine shows no significant skeletal or soft-tissue abnormalities and a normal width of the vertebral canal.

Following contrast injection, the myelogram documents unobstructed flow of the contrast medium and homogeneous opacification of the dural sac, which presents a normal diameter. The perimedullary arachnoid spaces are bilaterally symmetrical, and the spinal cord appears as a central filling defect of normal caliber. The thoracic root sheaths appear normal. The conus medullaris shows a normal configuration.

Interpretation

Normal thoracic myelogram with no evidence of a mass lesion or vascular malformation.

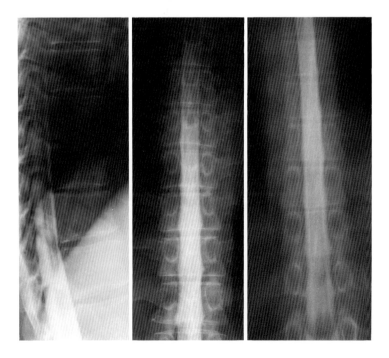

Checklist

Technique	• The spinal canal is punctured at the L2/L3 level, usually with the patient in lateral decubitus
	• With a slight head-down tilt (and initial fluoroscopic control to exclude epidural injection), ca. 10 mL of contrast medium (usually nonionic and usually more dense than for lumbar myelography) is injected within 30 s
	• The patient is immediately moved to a supine position following the injection
	• Spot films are taken at three levels under fluoroscopic control
	• If there is a block due to kyphosis, the head-down tilt may be increased or the patient moved to a supine position
	• Supine tomograms are obtained if small intramedullary lesions are suspected (e.g., angioma, dural fistula)
Plain radiograph	• Vertebral bodies (number, shape, structure, contours)
	• Spinal canal (smooth contours, width, see below)
	• Soft tissues (calcifications, swelling?)
Myelogram, opacification	• Homogeneous, no filling defects or voids
	• No block to the flow of contrast medium
	• No indentation of the dural sac
	• No tortuous tubular structures (e.g., veins)
Shape	• *Dural sac:*
	— Tubular shape conforming to the spinal canal
	— Central position (equal on both sides, no displacement)
	— Caliber
	— No intradural lesion (filling defect)
	— No extrinsic compression
	• *Spinal cord:*
	– Centered in the spinal canal
	— No intramedullary expansion, no narrowing
	— No extrinsic cord deformation (e.g., wavy contour)
	— Symmetrical origins of root sheaths
	• *Conus medullaris:*
	— Variable termination (usually at the L1/L2 level)
	— Caliber (no expansion)
	— Symmetrical contrast flow around the conus
Contours	• Smooth, sharply defined contours of dural sac and lateral root sheath margins
	• No contour defects (e.g., bandlike)

Lumbar Myelography

A lumbar puncture is performed, and 10 mL of nonionic contrast medium is injected into the spinal subarachnoid space. Radiographs are then obtained under fluoroscopic control.

The preliminary plain radiograph of the lumbar spine shows no significant skeletal or soft-tissue abnormalities and a normal width of the vertebral canal.

Following contrast injection, the myelogram documents unobstructed flow of the contrast medium and homogeneous opacification of the dural sac, which presents a normal shape and diameter. In the supine and head-down positions, the conus medullaris appears as a filling defect of normal caliber. The tapered, conical termination of the dural sac occurs at a normal level within the sacral canal. The lumbar and sacral root sheaths are bilaterally symmetrical in the PA and oblique projections and show no shortening or expansion. The contours of the dural sac and spinal roots are sharply defined.

Interpretation

The spinal canal, roots, and root sheaths in the lumbar region have a normal myelographic appearance.

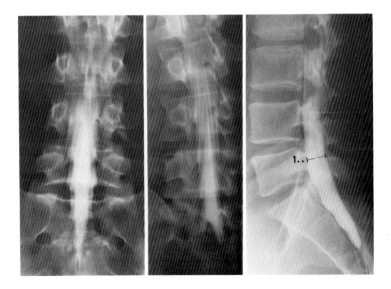

Checklist

Technique	• The spinal canal is punctured at the L3/L4 or L4/L5 level, usually with the patient in lateral decubitus
	• With a slight head-up tilt (and initial fluoroscopic control to exclude epidural injection), ca. 10 mL of contrast medium (usually nonionic) is injected over about a 1-minute period
	• Films: PA (prone position due to anterolateral emergence of the roots), lateral, and oblique (supine position); functional views may also be obtained
Plain radiograph	• Vertebral bodies (number, shape, structure, contours)
	• Spinal canal (smooth contours, width)
	• Soft tissues (calcifications, swelling?)
Myelogram, opacification	• Homogeneous, no filling defects or voids
	• No block to the flow of contrast medium
	• No indentation of the dural sac
Shape	• *Dural sac:*
	– Tubular shape conforming to the spinal canal
	– Central position (no displacement)
	– Caliber (see below)
	• *Conus medullaris* (in supine and head-down position):
	– Variable termination (see below)
	– Caliber (no expansion)
	– Symmetrical contrast flow around the conus
	• No expansion, constriction, or deformation (e.g., wavy contours)
	• Symmetrical origins of root sheaths (the higher their origin, the more vertical their course)
	• Root sheaths: length (equal on both sides), no cutoff, no splaying
	• Root cysts as normal variant?
Contours	• Smooth, sharply defined contours of dural sac and lateral root sheath margins
	• No contour defects (e.g., bandlike)
	• No double contours

Important Data

Dural sac:
1. Sagittal diameter > than 15 mm
Terminates at mid-sacral level
Conus medullaris terminates ca. at L1/L2 level

Bipedal Lymphangiography and Lymphadenography

Patent blue dye (0.5 mL) mixed with local anesthetic is injected subcutaneously into two interdigital spaces of each foot, the dye-labeled lymph vessels are exposed on the dorsum of the foot, and a total of 8 mL of Lipiodol is injected into the exposed lymph vessels on each side. The opacified lymph vessels demonstrate a normal course and caliber, and the lymphatic pathways can be traced into the thoracic duct. There is no evidence of collateral channels.

Films taken 24 hours after the injection show complete clearing of the lymph vessels. All the nodal groups visualized with this technique are opacified and are normal in size, shape, and structure.

Interpretation

The visualized lymph vessels and lymph nodes appear normal.

Checklist

Technique (e.g.)	• 0.5 mL of patent blue dye (mixed with local anesthetic) is injected subcutaneously into each of the interdigital spaces I/II and III/IV
	• The labeled lymph vessels are exposed on the dorsum of the foot
	• 8 mL of lipiodol is injected into the vessels on each side
	• Radiographs are taken before contrast injection, immediately after contrast injection, and at 24 hours postinjection (low pelvic AP view, AP abdominal, left and right oblique, AP thoracic)
Plain abdominal radiograph	• Spinal alignment (scoliosis, anomaly, etc.)
	• No calcifications
	• No soft-tissue densities (mass effect?)
Filling phase	• Opacification of all lymphatic pathways (femoral, inguinal, iliac, lumbar, thoracic)
	• Termination of the thoracic duct at the junction of the left subclavian and internal jugular veins
	• Normal caliber (see below) (compare with contralateral lymph pathways)
	• No circumscribed displacement
	• No cutoff of contrast column in lymph vessels
	• No abnormal collaterals
Storage phase	• Visualization of all nodal groups (prefascial and subfascial, inguinal, external and common iliac, lumbar)
	• Opacification: harmonious, granular to reticular pattern, finely stippled
	• Shape: bean-shaped, ovoid, round
	• Size: variable, compare with other lymph nodes
	• No filling defects
	• No rarefaction of nodal structure
Follow-up chest film	• Oil embolism, pneumonia?

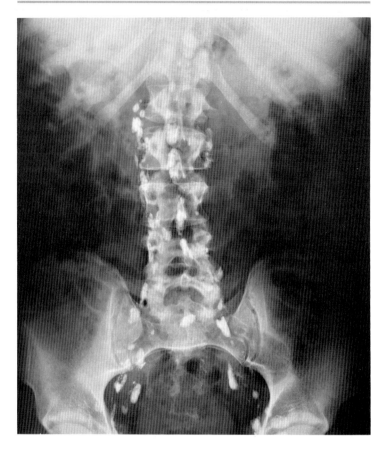

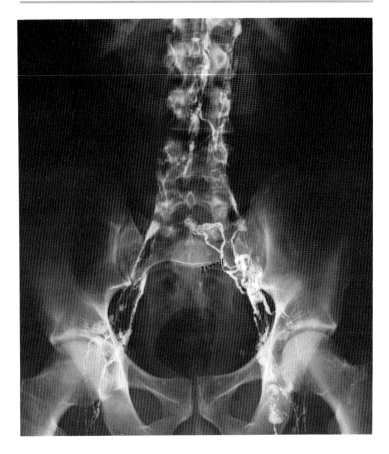

Important Data

1. Diameter of lymphatic pathways = 1–4 mm

Bronchography

Following topical anesthesia of the upper airways, a flexible rubber Ch 16 catheter is passed successively into the individual lobar bronchi of the lung, and a total of 8 mL of a water-soluble contrast material is injected.

This study demonstrates a normal course and distribution of the bronchial system to the level of the terminal branches. The bronchi are normal in caliber and have smooth, sharply defined walls. There is no evidence of filling defects.

The follow-up chest film shows no abnormal sites of contrast retention.

Interpretation

Normal bronchogram.

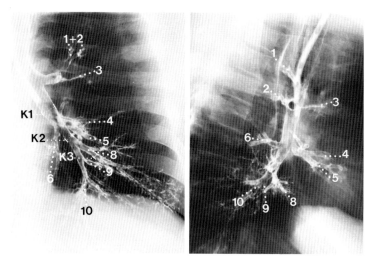

Important Data

Calibers:
Main bronchus K_1 = 11–17 mm
Secondary bronchus K_2 = 5–7 mm
Tertiary bronchus K_3 = 3–5 mm
Bifurcation angle = 55–64°

Checklist

Technique (e. g.)	• Topical anesthesia of the nasopharynx and trachea
	• A flexible rubber Ch 13–18 catheter is passed into the main bronchus and lobar bronchi, and about 8 mL of a water-soluble contrast material is injected (avoid overinjection!)

Bronchus, anatomy

Right:

- Upper lobe:
  1. Apical segmental bronchus
  2. Posterior seg. br.
  3. Anterior seg. br.
- Middle lobe:
  4. Lateral seg. br.
  5. Medial seg. br.
- Lower lobe:
  6. Apical seg. br.
  7. Cardiac seg. br.
  8. Anterobasal seg. br.
  9. Laterobasal seg. br.
  10. Posterobasal seg. br.

Left:

- Upper lobe:
  1.+2. Apicoposterior seg. br.
  3. Anterior seg. br.
  4. Superior seg. br. (lingula)
  5. Inferior seg. br. (lingula)
- Lower lobe:
  6. Apical seg. br.
  8. Anterobasal seg. br.
  9. Laterobasal seg. br.
  10. Posterobasal seg. br.

Shape
- Course (dichotomous distribution)
- Caliber (see below): harmonious taper
- Intricate structure
- No sacciform or cylindrical protrusions

Lumen
- Visualized to the level of the terminal branches
- No cutoff of contrast column
- No intraluminal filling defect
- No extraluminal impressions
- No displacement

Contours
- Smooth and sharp

Follow-up chest film
- No abnormal contrast pooling in PA chest film (ca. 2 hours postinjection)

Parotid Sialography

The plain radiograph demonstrates a normal bone structure of the mandible and normal-appearing soft tissues with no swelling or calcifications.

A probe is inserted into the excretory duct of the parotid gland. A thin catheter is inserted for a distance of about 1 cm, and a total of 1.5 mL of iodinated contrast medium is injected.

The excretory duct of the gland occupies a normal position and has a normal caliber and length. It shows a normal dendritic pattern of division into side branches. The duct system is normal in its course and extent and has smooth wall contours. There is no obstruction of contrast drainage from the duct system.

Interpretation

The duct system of the parotid gland appears normal.

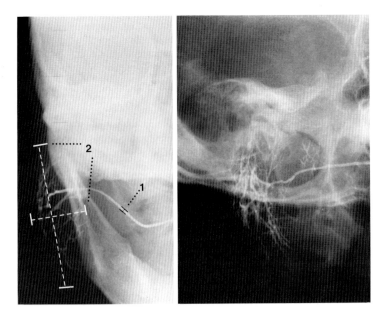

Checklist

Plain radiograph	• Mandible: shape, size, position, bone structure, contours
	• Soft tissues show no swelling or calcifications
Technique	• A probe is inserted into the excretory duct of the parotid gland
	• The duct is dilated as required
	• A catheter (ca. 2 Ch) is advanced about 1 cm into the duct
	• 1.5 mL of iodinated contrast medium (usually 60%) is injected
Duct system	• Shape
	• Position
	• Caliber (see below)
	• Length (variable)
	• Dendritic division into side branches
	• No duct cutoff
	• No duct displacement
	• Smooth, sharp delineation of the duct system
	• No circumscribed filling defects or niches
	• No ectasia
Parenchyma	• Shape
	• Size (see below; estimated from the extent of the duct system)
	• Unobstructed drainage of contrast medium (see below)

Important Data

1. *Duct caliber:* 0.8–3.2 mm. Maximum right–left difference = 0.7 mm
2. *Size of gland:* 10–20 cm^2. Maximum right–left difference = 2.5 cm^2

Contrast drainage: usually at 5 minutes p.i.

Hysterosalpingography

Preliminary fluoroscopy demonstrates normal skeletal structures and soft tissues of the lesser pelvis. There are no abnormal calcifications or radiopaque foreign bodies. A cannula is placed against the cervical os, and a total of 7 mL of iodinated contrast medium is injected.

The study demonstrates a smooth-bordered cervical canal of normal length and diameter. The uterine cavity is normally positioned, and the contrast medium fills it without obstruction. The cavity displays smooth contours, a normal shape, and normal distensibility with no filling defects. The uterine tubes are symmetrically disposed, have normal diameters, and show unobstructed filling. The mucosal relief of the ampullary portions is unremarkable. There are no filling defects or persistent niches. There is normal, bilateral spillage of contrast material into the peritoneal cavity.

Interpretation

Normal hysterosalpingogram.

Checklist

Fluoroscopic findings
- Lesser pelvis:
  - Skeleton (shape, size, symmetry, structure, contours)
  - Soft tissues (no increased soft-tissue densities)
- No calcifications (ovary, uterus, bladder)
- No radiopaque foreign bodies

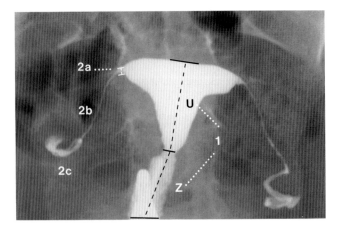

Technique	• A cervical cannula is placed against the external os under vision
	• A total of about 7 mL contrast medium is injected under fluoroscopic control (PA views, perhaps with side elevated)
	(Delayed films may be obtained at 30 minutes)
Uterus	• Cervical canal:
	— Length (see below)
	— Smooth or "feathery" pattern
	• Uterine cavity:
	— Position (central, retroflexion or anteflexion)
	— Unobstructed filling
	— Normal, harmonious distensibility
	— Normal shape (see below), smooth concavity of uterine sidewalls
	— Wall contours (smooth, sharp)
	— No intravasation of contrast material
	— No sinus tracts
Uterine tubes	• Unobstructed contrast drainage
	• Bilateral symmetry of tubes
	• Four parts (intramural part, isthmus, ampulla, infundibulum)
	• Normal diameter (see below)
	• Sometimes visible: longitudinal folds of mucosa in the tubal ampullae
	• No filling defects or niches
	• Normal mobility (if evaluated)
Peritoneal cavity	• Unobstructed bilateral contrast spillage from the uterine tubes (delayed films at 30 minutes, taken only in exceptional cases, should show emptying of the uterine cavity and tubes)
Contours	• Visible outer contours of the ovary and uterus (ovaries bilaterally symmetrical, uterus centered on the midline)

Important Data

1. Ratio of cervical (z) length to length of uterine cavity (U) = 3:4 (usually can be evaluated only on drainage film)
2. Tubal dimensions:
   (**a**) Intramural part = 1–2.5 mm in diameter
   (**b**) Isthmus = variable length, filamentous
   (**c**) Ampulla = widest (ca. 5–8 mm) and longest part (ca. 6–8 cm)

Depression of uterine fundus: up to 1 cm = normal, 1.5–2 cm = arcuate uterus, more than 2 cm = bicornuate uterus

Galactography

A cannula is inserted into the secreting milk duct. A water-soluble iodinated contrast material is injected, and radiographs of the breast are obtained in two projections.

The opacified milk duct appears normal in its shape, position, and caliber. It displays a normal branching pattern and unremarkable wall contours. The acini show a normal arrangement and morphology.

Interpretation

The duct system of the examined breast appears normal.

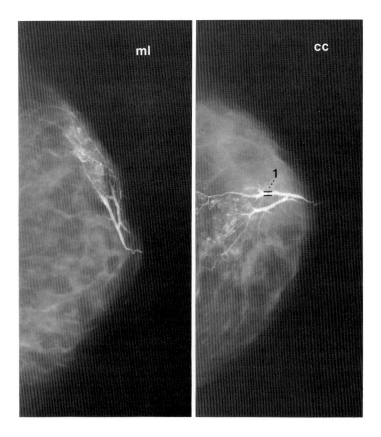

Checklist

Technique
- The nipple area is cleaned, and compression is applied to the breast until moisture appears at the orifice of the secreting milk duct
- The milk duct is dilated with a probe as required
- A cannula (e.g., lacrimal) or plastic tube is inserted
- The nipple is pulled upward
- 1–3 mL of a water-soluble iodinated contrast material (50%, without air!) is injected, according to pain tolerance
- The cannula is removed, and the duct orifice is occluded (a spray dressing may be used)
- Biplane mammograms are obtained in the craniocaudal (cc) and mediolateral (ml) projections

Duct system
- Shape
- Position
- Caliber (see below)
- Length (variable)
- Dendritic division into side branches
- No duct obstruction (cutoff)
- No duct displacement
- Smooth, sharp wall contours
- No circumscribed filling defects or niches
- No ectasia
- No fistulae

Mammary lobules
- Shape
- Position
- Size
- No displacement or impression
- No filling defects or ectasia
- No microcysts

Important Data

1. *Caliber of milk duct:* less than 3 mm

Index